Granulocyte Serology
A Clinical and Laboratory Guide

JEFFREY McCULLOUGH, MD

Professor
Department of Laboratory Medicine
  and Pathology
University of Minnesota Medical
  School
Minneapolis, Minnesota

Director
University of Minnesota Hospital
  Blood Bank
Minneapolis, Minnesota

Director
St Paul Regional Red Cross Blood
  Services
St Paul, Minnesota

CYNTHIA PRESS, MT(ASCP)

Consultant
St Paul Regional Red Cross Blood
  Services
St Paul, Minnesota

MARY CLAY, MT(ASCP)

Associate Scientist
Department of Laboratory Medicine
  and Pathology
University of Minnesota Medical
  School
Minneapolis, Minnesota

WILLIAM KLINE, MS, MT(ASCP)SBB

Director of Technical Services
St Paul Regional Red Cross Blood
  Services
St Paul, Minnesota

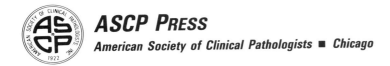

ASCP PRESS
American Society of Clinical Pathologists ■ Chicago

Cover: Scanning electron micrograph of human blood
granulocytes.
Cover photo courtesy of: Sally L Palm, PhD

Library of Congress Cataloging-in-Publication Data

Granulocyte serology.

  Includes bibliographies and index.
  1. Granulocyte antigens—Analysis. I. McCullough,
Jeffrey J. [DNLM: 1. Blood Transfusion. 2. Granulocytes.
3. Serology—methods.   WH 200 G7644]
QR186.6.G73G73   1988   616.07'92   87-19264
ISBN 0-89189-254-0

93 92 91 90 89   5 4 3 2 1

PRINTED IN THE UNITED STATES OF AMERICA

Contents

Part Two Laboratory Practice

List of Procedures

List of Figures

List of Tables

Preface

A quarter of a century has elapsed since the recognition of the first granulocyte-specific antigen and the subsequent development of granulocyte serology. Our experience in the field has reflected its evolution from an immunologic curiosity to a recognized component of immunohematology.

In recent years, we have found the medical community to be increasingly aware of the impact of granulocyte antibodies in various clinical situations and eager to obtain prompt, relevant laboratory data regarding their presence. Reflecting this clinical interest, our assistance has been increasingly solicited in establishing testing programs and obtaining antisera, as well as in providing serologic testing and clinical interpretation. These inquiries emphasized that a consolidated source of information in this field was no more available today than it was when we began the development of our granulocyte serology program.

We have therefore attempted to consolidate our experiences in a format useful to both laboratories providing granulocyte serologic services and clinicians interested in utilizing such services. Theoretical foundations as well as practical applications are included for this purpose. We hope that the extensive bibliography and the liberal use of diagrammatic, tabular, and pictorial presentations will enhance this book's value as a reference.

Further understanding of granulocyte antigens and antibodies will certainly be aided by some standardization of techniques and approaches, in addition to increased exchange of information and antisera. It is our hope that this book will encourage the continued development of granulocyte serology.

Acknowledgments

The development and growth of our granulocyte serology program has been greatly facilitated by the training and assistance provided to us by the following individuals, to whom we express our sincere appreciation: Dr Parviz Lalezari, Dr John S Thompson, Dr Paul Terasaki, Dr Ian Drew, Dr Frans Claas, Dr Jon van Rood, Dr Albert von dem Borne, and Dr Paul Engelfriet. And, we take this opportunity to thank Dr Harry Jacob and Dr Gregory Vercellotti for providing the cytoplast methodology adopted in our lab.

We would like to acknowledge the invaluable assistance of Anne Gay, Catherine Maddox, David Olson, Dr Sylvia Gunawan, and Dr Karen Richards, who contributed, revised, and reviewed the details and/or diagrams of the laboratory procedures included in the Methods section. We also give our special thanks to Dr Hannis Thompson, who provided the material for the section on the Systematic Approach to the Diagnosis of Neutropenia, and to Dr Sally L Palm who provided the cover micrograph.

We particularly thank Judy Johns, Pat Derks, Penny Milne, Marlene Brave, and Pat Swenson for secretarial work; the staff of the University of Minnesota Biomedical Graphics Department for preparing the diagrams and photographs; and Joshua Weikersheimer and the staff of the ASCP Press for their generous assistance and support during the preparation of this material for publication.

Finally, we are greatly indebted to the numerous individuals in medical centers throughout the world for their confidence and cooperation as shown by the referral of specimens, without which we would have been unable to develop our granulocyte serology program.

Part I

Clinical Considerations

Chapter 1

Historical Perspectives on Granulocyte Serology

Most work with blood cell antigens has involved erythrocytes, probably because these were the most common and readily available blood cells, and because most transfusions were of red blood cells. In recent decades, studies of antigens of other blood cells and tissues have also paralleled their application to transfusion and transplantation. However, even in the early years of this century, some investigators directed their attention to leukocytes. In 1926 Doan[1] observed that the sera of some patients caused agglutination of leukocytes from other individuals. Initially it was not clear whether this agglutination represented a true antibody-antigen reaction, because of the tendency of leukocyte suspensions to spontaneously clump and the panagglutinating nature of the sera. Later studies using improved leukoagglutination techniques established that these were true antibody-antigen reactions.

Further interest in leukocyte serology was stimulated by a series of publications in the 1950s. These described the detection of leukoagglutinins in the sera of polytransfused persons,[2,3] the occurrence of white cell agglutinins in response to fetomaternal immunization,[4,5] drug-related leukocyte antibodies,[6] and the role of leukocyte antibodies in febrile transfusion reactions.[7] However, work with these leukocyte antibodies progressed slowly due to the technical difficulties of standardizing assays and the variability of results inherent in the leukoagglutination method. These problems were overcome by the development of the microlymphocytotoxicity test.[8] However, this shifted much of the leukocyte antibody work to the lymphocyte, and the use of this test system to define the human leukocyte antigen (HLA) system is well known. A few investigators continued to use leukoagglutination techniques to work with granulocyte serology. In the 1960s, Lalezari used an improved granulocyte agglutination technique to study neutropenic newborns, leading to the discovery of a series of antigens that are limited to neutrophils.[9-13] Subsequent studies of granulocyte antigen and antibody systems have established their genetic polymorphism and revealed clinical situations analogous to those defined by red blood cell serology. Antibodies directed against granulocyte antigens have been implicated in neonatal neutropenia, autoimmune neutropenia, febrile transfusion reactions, and severe transfusion reactions associated with pulmonary infiltrates.

While the extent of knowledge of granulocyte serology does not yet approach that of the red blood cell or HLA systems, continued interest through the years has established a definite role for studies of granulocyte antigens and antibodies. Current knowledge has demonstrated distinct clinical applications, and future studies promise insight into relationships between granulocyte antigens and cellular function.

Chapter 2

Methods for Detection of Granulocyte Antibodies

The study of granulocyte antibodies has important clinical relevance. Antibodies have been shown to play important roles in alloimmune neonatal neutropenia,[14-18] autoimmune neutropenias,[19-22] transfusion reactions,[7,23] and the ability of granulocytes to localize at the sites of infection.[24,25] There are also reports showing that granulocyte antibodies can affect the normal function of granulocytes in vitro.[26-28]

Working with granulocytes requires both an understanding of their intrinsic physiologic composition and technical finesse. Unlike red blood cells, which are relatively easy to test in vitro, granulocytes are nucleated cells containing cytoplasm filled with lysosomal granules and surrounded by a fluid membrane that makes them fragile and sensitive to collection, processing, and storage conditions. These properties are essential to their basic phagocytic function but can easily contribute to autolysis and spontaneous aggregation when the cells are damaged. Therefore, for assays that require viable and functional granulocytes, it is necessary to minimize their exposure to glass surfaces, high ($> 500 \times$ g) gravitational forces, low ($< 18°C$) and high ($> 37°C$) temperatures, and excessive manipulation. Modifications in techniques or reagents from the proven methods may render them ineffective due to inadvertent granulocyte damage. With regard to granulocyte serologic assays, it is sometimes helpful to observe the following axiom: There is no need to fix what isn't broken.

Laboratory approaches for the detection of granulocyte antibodies require procedures that are accurate, reproducible, and practical. Although numerous granulocyte serologic assays have been described, not all fulfill all of these criteria. The following discussion of methods will focus on their capabilities for detection of granulocyte antigens and antibodies, as well as for implementation in the laboratory. In addition to the assay used, detection of antibodies or antigens may also depend on the concentration of target cells, the target cell antigen density, and the concentration and immunoglobulin class and/or subclass of the antibody in question. The presently known granulocyte antigen systems have been "serologically defined" using different assays that are, in general, not interchangeable or directly comparable. Therefore, the successful detection of granulocyte antibodies often requires use of more than one method. As performance of multiple assays may not be feasible, a more practical approach would be utilizing one or two basic screening methods and/or referring specimens to specialized laboratories for evaluation.

Numerous serologic techniques have been developed for the detection of granulocyte antibodies. Most may be categorized by their mode of detection: (1) direct agglutination of cells, (2) complement-dependent cytotoxicity, (3) cell-bound immunoglobulin, and (4) cell-mediated granulocytotoxicity (Table 2–1). Some of these assays have been developed to detect antibodies associated with specific clinical disorders and have not been widely applied. There-

Table 2–1.	Granulocyte Antibody Detection Methods	
Category	Specific Technique	Reference
Agglutination	Granulocyte microagglutination	29,56
	Microcapillary agglutination	63
Complement-dependent cytotoxicity	Granulocytotoxicity	70,78
	Double fluorochromasia	63,76
Immunoglobulin binding	Immunofluorescence	20
	Staphylococcal protein A	87,91,92
	Avidin-biotin immunoassay	100
	Enzyme-linked immunosorbent assay	106
	Opsonic assay	26
	Antiglobulin consumption	94
	Radiolabeled anti-C3	107
	Radiolabeled antiglobulin	108
	Fab-anti-Fab	121,369
Functional assay	Inhibition of granulocyte phagocytosis	118
	Cell elasticity technique	119
	Inhibition of myeloid maturation	117
Cell-mediated cytotoxicity	Antibody-dependent lymphocyte-mediated granulocytotoxicity	109,115

fore, the relationships of the results of these tests to a variety of clinical situations are not well established.[29] Although many methods exist, no single technique has thus far been shown to consistently detect all clinically relevant granulocyte antibodies.

Preparation of Pure Granulocyte Suspensions

Most assays for granulocyte antibody detection require isolation of purified granulocytes for target antigens. One difficulty of early granulocyte serologic studies was the lack of such pure granulocyte preparations. Results were affected by contaminating red blood cells, platelets, and lymphocytes in the cell suspension. Defibrination,[30] differential centrifugation,[31] gum acacia,[32] dextran,[33] polyvinylpyrrolidone (PVP),[9] hexadimethrine bromide (polybrene),[31] lectins,[34] and anti-A,B[34] were all used at various times in attempts to produce enriched granulocyte suspensions. None of these methods proved totally satisfactory.

The isolation of pure cell populations from human peripheral blood was simplified with the introduction in 1968 of Boyum's Ficoll-Isopaque gradient technique.[35] Density gradient centrifugation employing Ficoll or Percoll gradients is now the most widely used approach for the isolation and purification of granulocytes for serologic testing. Numerous publications describe the recovery, purity, functional integrity, and activity of isolated granulocytes.[36–39]

Ficoll Gradients

Ficoll is a hydrophilic sucrose polymer of high molecular weight (mol wt 400,000) that must be deionized and dehydrated prior to gradient preparation. Ficoll solutions are highly viscous, but with the addition of Isopaque (sodium metrizoate) or Hypaque (sodium diatrizoate) specific densities can be prepared that are very suitable for cell separation.

Initially, granulocytes were isolated using single gradient techniques. The granulocytes were contained in the erythrocyte pellet, and it required hypotonic lysis to rid the granulocytes of red blood cells. However, the use of lysing agents in granulocyte preparation procedures has been an issue. Treatment of human lymphocytes with ammonium chloride to remove contaminating red blood cells has been shown to markedly reduce their cytotoxic effector cell activity in antibody-dependent cell-mediated cytotoxicity (ADCC) tests.[40] Loss of granulocyte function has been reported when granulocytes were exposed to hypotonic solutions with osmolalities less than 150 mosm.[41]

This potential problem was circumvented by English and Anderson's introduction of a discontinuous Ficoll-Hypaque gradient for simultaneous separation of mononuclear leukocytes, neutrophils, and erythrocytes.[36] We have used this procedure with the substitution of leukocyte-rich plasma for diluted whole blood to obtain granulocyte suspensions that are greater than 90% pure, eliminating the need for hypotonic lysis of red blood cells.[29] A schematic description of this gradient is shown in Figure 2–1. Ficoll-Hypaque solutions may be prepared or purchased commercially in such solutions as Histopaque-1.077 and -1.119 (Sigma Chemical Company). Unless large quantities are needed, it is usu-

---

Figure 2–1.

Diagrammatic isolation of mononuclear leukocytes (Layer 1), polymorphonuclear leukocytes (Layer 2), and erythrocytes (Layer 3) by centrifugation of leukocyte-rich plasma on a discontinuous gradient of Ficoll-Hypaque (1,650 × g for 15 minutes) or Percoll (400 × g for 20 minutes).

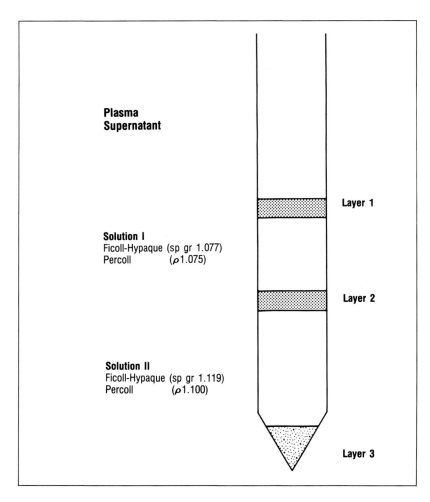

Plasma
Supernatant

Layer 1

Solution I
Ficoll-Hypaque (sp gr 1.077)
Percoll   (ρ1.075)

Layer 2

Solution II
Ficoll-Hypaque (sp gr 1.119)
Percoll   (ρ1.100)

Layer 3

ally more cost-efficient to purchase the prepared product. Preparation of the gradient solutions can be time-consuming, and standardization occasionally involves manipulations that are more magical than scientific in nature.

Major criticisms of Ficoll gradients focus on their limited ability for heterogenous cell separations,[42] their hypertonic osmolarity,[42] and their possible adverse effect on the metabolism of certain leukocytes.[43-47] The development of Percoll was designed to overcome these problems.

Percoll Gradients

Percoll consists of 15 to 30 nm colloidal silica particles that have been coated with polyvinylpyrrolidone. Percoll solutions have a low viscosity, can be made iso-osmolar, and have been found to be nontoxic to cells.[44,46] Although a major advantage of this separation medium is its ability to form self-generated gradients when centrifuged at high forces (eg, 30,000 × g) in an angle-head rotor, it is possible to prepare discontinuous, continuous linear, and continuous nonlinear gradients with bench-top centrifuges utilizing lower (eg, 400 × g) forces. In addition, formulas used for the preparation of working solutions from stock solutions and the stability of stock Percoll solutions facilitate the standardization of these gradients. A schematic diagram illustrating the composition of the discontinuous Percoll gradient we have used for the isolation of pure granulocytes is shown in Figure 2–1.

Although granulocytes isolated on Percoll gradients have demonstrated good recovery and have been shown to be pure, viable, and functionally active,[48,49] the initial higher cost of Percoll reagents compared to Ficoll products tends to discourage their use for routine granulocyte preparations.

Comparison of Gradient Methods

To compare the use of these two gradient products for granulocyte serology testing, we first measured the percentage recovery and purity of granulocyte suspensions isolated from leukocyte-rich plasma and centrifuged on discontinuous gradients of Ficoll-Hypaque and Percoll. As shown in Table 2–2, Percoll gradients produced a slightly better yield and recovery of granulocytes. The granulocyte suspensions were of comparable purity, with both gradients producing granulocyte suspensions that were nearly platelet-free (2.6 platelets per 100 granulocytes). It has been shown that the presence of one platelet per granulocyte in granulocyte suspensions used for in vitro testing can augment granulocyte aggregation.[50] Therefore, platelet contamination should be minimized.

Next, we evaluated the cost and time associated with the preparation of granulocytes from varying volumes of blood using both gradients in our laboratory (Table 2–3). The gradient price in-

Table 2–2. **Characteristics of Granulocytes Isolated Simultaneously on Discontinuous Ficoll-Hypaque and Percoll Gradients**

	n	Ficoll-Hypaque $\bar{x}$	Ficoll-Hypaque range	Percoll $\bar{x}$	Percoll range
Number of leukocytes applied per gradient ($\times 10^6$)	8	34.5	(17.6–55.8)	34.5	(17.6–55.8)
Number of granulocytes isolated ($\times 10^6$)*	8	17.6	(5.3–29.1)	19.2	(8.4–28.9)
Granulocyte recovery from LRP (%)	8	53.8	(23.2–87.7)	59.2	(34.0–84.6)
Composition of granulocyte suspension					
Granulocytes (%)	13	91.5	(86.6–97.7)	90.4	(78.0–97.7)
Mononuclear (%)	13	0.1	(0–0.2)	1.0	(0–4.3)
Red cells (%)	13	8.4	(2.3–13.3)	8.6	(1.7–21.7)
Number of platelets per 100 granulocytes	5	2.6	(1.9–3.7)	2.6	(1.8–3.9)

NOTE: Twenty-seven mL of EDTA blood was sedimented with 5 mL 1% methyl cellulose. The leukocyte rich plasma (LRP) was harvested and separated into two equal volumes for centrifugation on each gradient.

* Represents granulocytes obtained from LPR of 13.5 mL EDTA blood.

Table 2–3. **Cost and Time Analysis of Granulocytes Isolated on Discontinuous Ficoll-Hypaque and Percoll Gradients**

	Volume of Whole Blood Processed									
	14 mL		28 mL		42 mL		56 mL		70 mL	
Gradient	Cost ($)	Time (hrs)	Cost ($)	Time (hrs)	Cost ($)	Time (hrs)	Cost ($)	Time (hrs)	Cost ($)	Time (hrs)
Ficoll-Hypaque										
Ficoll solutions[a]	0.33		0.66		0.99		1.32		1.65	
Equipment[b]	0.41		0.82		1.23		1.64		2.05	
Total	0.74	1.5	1.48	1.6	2.22	1.7	2.96	1.8	3.70	1.9
Percoll										
Percoll solutions	0.80		0.80		0.80		0.80		0.80	
Equipment[b]	0.33		0.50		0.74		0.91		1.08	
Total	1.13	2.0	1.30	2.1	1.54	2.2	1.71	2.3	1.88	2.4

[a] Ficoll solutions prepared in our laboratory; not purchased as commercially prepared solutions.

[b] Includes reagents and disposable lab supplies used for the cell preparation and isolation procedure.

cluded only the cost of the separation solutions, reagents, and disposable lab supplies used solely for the cell separation procedure. Because of variable factors affecting the preparation of the gradient solutions, no attempt was made to include the cost of those supplies or technical time in this analysis. When granulocytes from 14 mL of blood were isolated on each gradient, the cost of the Ficoll cell preparation was approximately one third less than the cost of the Percoll cells ($0.74 and $1.13, respectively) (Table 2–3). However, because of the ability to load one Percoll gradient with as many as 1 to 2 × 10⁸ leukocytes,[49] the cost of processing granulocytes from more than 14 mL of blood is less expensive using Percoll gradients. It is not clear if Ficoll gradients can accommodate the high cell numbers that Percoll gradients are capable of handling. It takes approximately 1.5 hours to prepare granulocytes from 14 mL of blood on Ficoll gradients versus 2.0 hours on Percoll gradients. Each additional 14 mL of blood processed adds about six extra minutes of processing time, regardless of gradient product.

The pH and osmolality of solutions which comprise the Ficoll-Hypaque and Percoll gradients are shown in Table 2–4. The osmolalities of the Percoll solutions were nearly iso-osmolar. As previously noted, the heavier solution in the Ficoll gradient was hypertonic (514 mosm). Granulocytes isolated on Ficoll gradients are exposed to both acidic and hypertonic conditions. In contrast, Percoll has a very low buffering capacity and can be adjusted to pH 5.5–10.0, depending on the diluent used to make the stock Percoll solutions.

Finally, granulocytes isolated on each gradient were typed for the known granulocyte antigens using the granulocyte agglutination (GA) and granulocyte immunofluorescence (GIF) assays. In

Table 2–4.   **pH and Osmolality of Discontinuous Ficoll-Hypaque and Percoll Solutions**

Gradient	Solution No.	Osmolality mosm/kg/H₂O	pH
Ficoll-Hypaque	1 (1.077)[a]	300	5.8
	2 (1.119)[a]	514	6.4
Percoll	1 (1.075)[b]	309	8.0[c]
	2 (1.100)[b]	320	8.0[c]

[a] Specific gravity.

[b] Density.

[c] pH of Percoll solutions when Percoll stock solution is prepared with phosphate-buffered saline (pH 7.2) as the diluent.

the GA assay, there was no significant difference ($\chi^2 = 103.8$; $p < .001$) between the typing results of Percoll-separated versus Ficoll-separated granulocytes. However, in the GIF assay, granulocytes isolated on Percoll gradients demonstrated a high (41%) incidence of weak false positive typings compared with Ficoll granulocytes. This appeared to be due to an increase in nonspecific membrane fluorescence associated with Percoll-separated cells, possibly as a result of incomplete removal of Percoll particles from the granulocytes. Additional washing of cells might provide Percoll-prepared granulocytes that could be used in the GIF assay, but time delays and cell loss are limiting factors.

Granulocytes isolated on Ficoll gradients require less preparation time and contain less residual gradient solutions after washing than granulocytes separated with Percoll. Percoll gradients require less technical time for reagent preparation, are more reproducible from batch to batch, and are easier to standardize and quality-control. However, if large volumes of density gradient medium are not needed, the most efficient granulocyte isolation approach is the use of commercially prepared Ficoll-Hypaque solutions.

Detection of Circulating Antibodies

Granulocyte Agglutination

It is important to clarify the semantics associated with leukocyte terminology used in the 1950s and the corresponding current terminology used in granulocyte serology. HLA antibodies were initially investigated with an agglutination procedure using total leukocyte suspensions often contaminated with varying amounts of platelets and red blood cells.[51] This "leukoagglutination" technique was difficult to standardize partially because of the contaminating cells, and it gave variable results due to the tendency for leukocytes to clump nonspecifically. The development of the microlymphocytotoxicity test eliminated these problems for HLA testing.[52,53] Successful utilization of the agglutination procedure for granulocyte serology testing requires pure granulocyte suspensions isolated by density separation gradients. Hence, the term leukoagglutination does not refer to the "granulocyte agglutination" technique.

Using a macro granulocyte agglutination assay, Lalezari initially detected granulocyte-specific antibodies in the early 1960s.[10,54] His work established granulocyte agglutination as a reference procedure, which has been subsequently modified to use micro techniques.[55,56] Microagglutination tests as currently performed require fresh and viable granulocytes, utilize micro (1 to 5 μL) amounts of serum and cell suspensions, and are usually done in microtest plates under oil. The use of pure granulocyte suspensions and critical concentrations of EDTA have vastly improved the reproducibility of test reactions seen with this assay.[57,58]

Both IgM and IgG agglutinins can be detected with this procedure. In contrast to red blood cell agglutination, the primary mechanism responsible for granulocyte agglutination associated with IgG antibodies is not the same as that known to occur with red blood cells. Agglutination does not appear to be caused by cross-linking granulocytes via one antibody molecule Fab fragment attaching to one cell and the other Fab fragment binding to an adjacent cell. Agglutination results from neutrophil response to antibody stimulation, requires active cell participation, and is biphasic (Figure 2–2). The two phases have been designated as sensitization and agglutination.[9]

Figure 2–2.

Schematic representation of the granulocyte agglutination (GA) assay. **Sensitization phase:** *reaction of antibody with granulocyte membrane antigen resulting in activation of sensitized granulocytes.* **Agglutination phase:** *"activated" granulocytes form pseudopods, move toward each other to establish membrane contact, and thus form aggregates.*

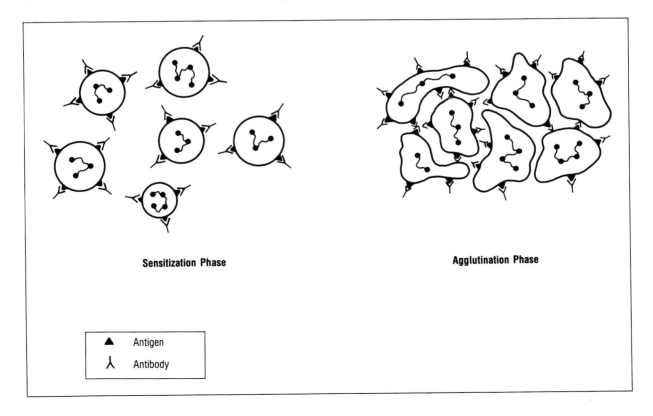

Sensitization Phase   Agglutination Phase

▲ Antigen

⅄ Antibody

The sensitization phase involves specific antibody reaction with cell surface antigens, does not lead to immediate agglutination, but does appear to "activate" the cells. During the agglutination phase the sensitized granulocytes form pseudopods and slowly move toward each other until membrane contact is established. It is not entirely clear whether agglutination is a result of changes in membrane-bound molecules that cause granulocytes to adhere to each other, or if they are cross-linked by antibodies bound via their Fab receptors to cell surface antigens on one granulocyte and via the Fc fragment of the bound antibody molecule to the specific Fc receptor of other granulocytes. Both phases are time- and temperature-dependent.[57] The procedure requires long incubation periods (4 to 6 hours) to allow cell movement to occur. The recommended incubation temperature of 30°C[56] allows for the detection of IgM and IgG antibodies and preserves cell viability, which can be significantly reduced by long incubation periods at 37°C.

The agglutination phase of the IgG antibody reaction process can be reversibly inhibited by incubation of the granulocytes at low temperatures, and irreversibly inhibited by heating the cells for 60 seconds at 56°C or by treatment of the cells with cytochalasin-B, an inhibitor of microfilament activity.[58,59] Conversely, IgM antibodies do demonstrate agglutination at low temperatures that are not inhibited by cytochalasin-B; thus, they most likely participate in direct agglutination by cross-linking granulocytes through antibody molecules.[60]

A popular modification of this assay uses a 2-hour incubation period at 37°C. However, this modification compromises its capability for the detection of granulocyte antibodies. Our experience with the method has shown that granulocyte viability can be affected by 2 hours of incubation at 37°C, and the amount of agglutination can be significantly reduced.

If done as specified, the assay is a reliable and reproducible technique for the detection of granulocyte agglutinins, and has been utilized in the identification of the following granulocyte antigens: NA1, NA2, NB1, NB2, NC1, ND1, NE1, and 9a.[57,61]

Thompson and Severson[62] have modified the granulocyte agglutination assay so it can be performed in microcapillary tubes and may be quantitated. The microcapillary agglutination assay (MCA) is more technically difficult to perform, appears to detect a broad range of IgG and IgM antibodies, is fast, is highly sensitive, and will detect granulocyte-specific antibodies.[63-65] Thompson et al have studied the association of antibodies detected in the MCA assay with clinical renal allograft function[66] and pulmonary hypersensitivity reactions induced by transfusion of non-HLA leukoagglutinins.[67] Smith and his colleagues[65] have found that this assay is useful in the detection of granulocyte antibodies in patients with autoimmune neutropenia.

Complement-Dependent Granulocyte Cytotoxicity

First utilized with lymphocytes, cytotoxicity methods have been modified and applied to the detection of complement-dependent granulocyte cytotoxins.[68,69] In these procedures, target granulocytes are first incubated with antisera to allow for binding of antibodies to cell surface antigens. Rabbit complement is then added to the test system. Antigen-antibody reactions capable of fixing and activating complement result in complement-mediated cell membrane damage. Damaged nonviable cells allow a vital dye, such as eosin or trypan blue, to penetrate the cell membrane. Nonviable cells can be distinguished from viable cells microscopically (Figure 2–3). Enzyme or cytochalasin-B treatment of cells has been used to enhance granulocytotoxin reactivity.[70,71]

Various modifications of the granulocyte cytotoxicity (GC) assay have been used by investigators attempting to identify a granulocyte antigen system solely by cytotoxins. Hasegawa et al[72] found several sera defining some granulocyte-specific antigens. His assay had maximum sensitivity at 5°C, and the immunoglobulin class detected by this assay was primarily IgM. Subsequent studies revealed that many of these sera contained cold-reacting autoantibodies. These antibodies are not generally believed to be clinically significant because they can be found in almost all normal sera.

Figure 2–3.

Schematic representation of the granulocyte cytotoxicity (GC) assay.

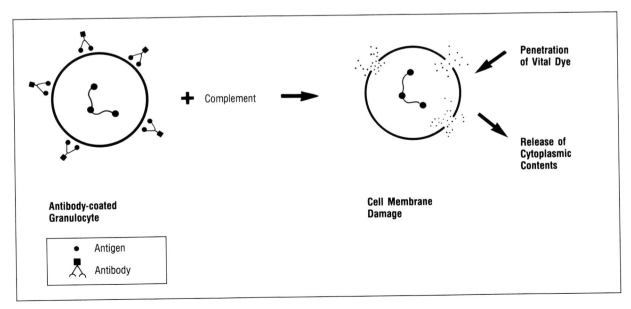

Antibody-coated Granulocyte

Complement

Penetration of Vital Dye

Release of Cytoplasmic Contents

Cell Membrane Damage

- Antigen
- Antibody

Using a different granulocytotoxicity assay, Caplan et al[70] found six sera that seemed to identify two alleles in a granulocyte antigen system, but their specificity for granulocytes was not reported. Korinkova et al[73] using both a modified granulocytotoxicity method and granulocyte agglutination assay, recently found nine sera that appeared to define three related groups of antigens.

The most recent cytotoxicity modification involves the double fluorochromatic technique of Takasugi.[74] It was concurrently described for platelet testing by Lizak and Grumet[75] and for granulocytes by Thompson and his associates.[76] Simultaneous visualization of the green viable cells and the red nonviable cells eliminated the difficulty often associated in reading dye exclusion reactions, and facilitated the use of automated instrumentation for tray reading. Using this assay, Thompson's group has reported three series of antigens: the first granulocyte-specific, the second found on both granulocytes and monocytes, and the third shared by granulocytes, monocytes, and endothelial cells.[63,76] Unfortunately, the paucity of sera remaining that identified these antigen groupings may preclude further work in this area. Blaschke et al[77] reported one case of a 29-year-old man with acquired agranulocytosis whose serum contained a granulocytotoxic autoantibody detected by their technique that disappeared upon disease resolution. The fluorochromatic GC method offers the advantage of both IgM and IgG antibody detection.[76]

There is now ample evidence that granulocytotoxicity detects a pattern of reactivity different from agglutination. However, the clinical significance and sensitivity of this test is still not clearly established. McCullough et al used a modified eosin dye exclusion assay[78,79] to study the clinical significance of the cytotoxic assay in patients receiving indium 111-labeled granulocytes. This study failed to detect any reduction in the intravascular recovery, half-life, or localization of granulocytes in patients with GC antibodies.[24] In addition to the questionable clinical significance of granulocytotoxicity results, the GC assay appears to offer no advantage in sensitivity. Preliminary results in Engelfriet's laboratory with a complement-binding anti-NA1 serum failed to show an increase in antibody titer when tested in the fluorochromasia cytotoxic assay versus the immunofluorescence assay using anti-C or anti-Ig.[59,60] Definition of antigen specificities by the granulocyte cytotoxicity technique awaits exchange of sera and interlaboratory comparison.

Immunoglobulin Binding

More than 15 years ago, Engelfriet and van Loghem reported a class of leukocyte antibodies which could not be detected by agglutination or cytotoxicity techniques.[33] Attempts have since been made to detect these antibodies on the surface of sensitized granulocytes using (1) secondary labeled antibodies, (2) tests which detect opsonic antibody activity, (3) tests which detect the ability of antibodies to interfere with granulocyte function, (4) inhibition assays, and (5) direct binding assays. Currently, the major thrust of activity directed at this type of antibody detection is focused on the use of secondary labeled antibodies in the immunofluorescence, staphylococcal protein A, and enzyme-linked immunosorbent assays. Thus, these assays will be discussed first.

Granulocyte Immunofluorescence (GIF) Utilization of a fluorescent "antiglobulin" technique for the study of leukopenic disorders was first approached by Calabresi and his co-workers in 1959.[80] Application of the technique for the detection of granulocyte antibodies was reported by Verheugt and his colleagues,[81,82] who used the assay to detect alloantibodies and autoantibodies that were both circulating and cell-bound.

Basically, immunoglobulins bound to the cell surface are detected by the addition of secondary antihuman immunoglobulins that are labeled with a fluorescent dye, eg, fluorescein isothiocyanate (FITC) or ethidium bromide (Figure 2–4). The reaction can be qualitatively graded according to the pattern and density of fluorescent spots on the cell surface, or the results can be more precisely quantitated by microfluorometry.[81]

Figure 2–4.

Schematic representation of the granulocyte immunofluorescence (GIF) assay.

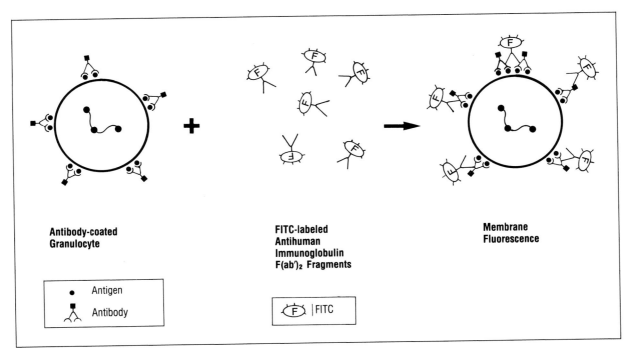

Antibody-coated
Granulocyte

• Antigen

⊼ Antibody

FITC-labeled
Antihuman
Immunoglobulin
F(ab')₂ Fragments

Ⓕ | FITC

Membrane
Fluorescence

Because of the high concentration of surface Fc receptors on granulocytes, a major problem was the fluorescence of granulocytes due to the nonspecific adherence of immunoglobulins to the cell membrane.[81] This was resolved by treating target cells with 1% paraformaldehyde (PFA) prior to incubation with test serum, and the use of $F(ab')_2$ fragments of conjugated antihuman immunoglobulins.[60] The exact mechanism by which PFA treatment reduces binding of monomeric immunoglobulins to granulocyte Fc receptors is not known. However, PFA treatment increases the negative charge of the cell membrane, and it has been suggested that this may stabilize the membrane and/or subsequently decrease the affinity of the Fc receptors for normal IgG.[58,81] Although PFA-treated cells are not viable, their membranes must be intact to prevent internalization of the FITC conjugate. This results in cytoplasmic fluorescence, indicating a damaged cell, which cannot be evaluated.

The original method of Verheugt required the use of 100 μL of serum and cell suspension for each test, which was done in a small microcentrifuge tube. Both the serum-cell quantity and tube manipulation created potential limitations for use in high-volume testing. Zaroulis and Jaramillo[83] introduced a modified procedure which reduced the serum and cell volumes to 10 μL, but the assay was still performed in microcentrifuge tubes, which were awkward to manipulate. The assay was transferred to microtiter plates by Press et al[84] with the use of 20 μL of serum and cell suspension. These micro modifications have greatly enhanced the practicality of the method for use in granulocyte serology programs.

Other than the agglutination assay, the GIF is the only assay shown to detect the known granulocyte-specific antigens NA1, NA2, NB1, NC1, ND1, and NE1.[81] However, NB2 and 9a, which have been reported to be closely associated or identical,[61] are nonreactive in the GIF test. The reason for this is not known. PFA treatment of the cells does not destroy the antigen, as shown by absorption studies.[81] It has been speculated that the avidity of the antibody binding is low; thus, disassociation of the antibody from the granulocyte surface may occur during the washing steps of the GIF procedure.[81]

Certain fluorescent labeling patterns may be associated with different types of antibodies. Most granulocyte-specific antibodies will have a fairly diffuse or homogeneous labeling pattern that can also appear as a fluorescent ring around the cell in the case of high-titer antibodies. However, anti-NB1 characteristically exhibits a mixed-field pattern ranging from negative to strong fluorescence.[59] We have seen some sera containing immune complexes which display large, bright fluorescent spots on the cell membranes.

Staphylococcal Protein A (SPA) SPA, a major cell wall component of most strains of *Staphylococcus aureus*, has an extraordinary affinity for IgG immunoglobulin, which makes it an attractive immunological probe for the detection of cell-surface–bound IgG.[85] The molecule contains four tyrosine residues that are easily radioiodinated,[85,86] or it can be labeled with FITC.[87] SPA exhibits the following binding properties: (1) binds specifically to the Fc portion of IgG; (2) binds only to IgG subclasses 1, 2, and 4; (3) fails to bind to IgG3; (4) may bind to a limited degree with IgM[85,88] (Figure 2–5). A sandwich technique in which anti-IgM or anti-C components are first reacted with the sensitized cells prior to the addition of SPA, expands the utility of the assay.[89] Because SPA appears to provide a sensitive quantitative approach to the detection of indirect or direct granulocyte antibody binding, much interest has been directed to its use.

Introduced by McCallister and co-workers,[87] the assay was used to study granulocyte antibodies in the serum of patients with alloimmune and autoimmune neutropenia. This initial study not only indicated the increased sensitivity of the assay compared to opsonic antibody testing, it also demonstrated the mobilization of surface antigens into polar-capped pseudopodia by SPA. Harmon's group[90]

Figure 2–5.

Schematic representation of the staphylococcal protein A (SPA) assay.

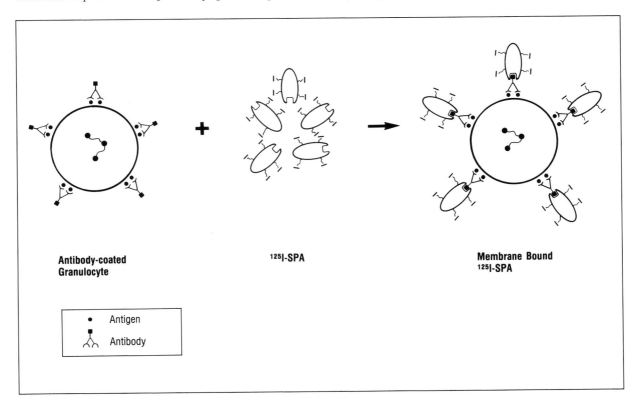

Antibody-coated Granulocyte

125I-SPA

Membrane Bound 125I-SPA

| • | Antigen |
| Y | Antibody |

then developed a slide test for the detection of direct or indirect granulocyte antibodies by killed Cowan 1 staphylococci containing protein A. This approach had three major practical advantages. First, a panel of cells could be fixed on glass slides and stored in buffer for up to 3 weeks. Second, even neutropenic patients could provide blood smears with a few granulocytes present for evaluation. And third, the application of staphylococcal bacteria directly to the fixed cells allowed visualization of the cells participating in SPA binding and the surface topography of antibody-antigen reactions. Harmon et al went on to extend the slide test to detect complement components on neutrophils, and demonstrated that C3 without IgG may be responsible for neutrophil destruction in some cases of immune neutropenia.[91]

A micro modification of McCallister's original method was recently reported by Lazar et al.[92] The use of microtiter trays, the reduced serum and cell volume, and the use of fixed cells that can be stored for up to 48 hours enhance the use of this assay for large-scale serum screening.

Although the SPA assay cannot discriminate between alloimmune and autoimmune processes, the assay has been reported to distinguish immune neutropenia from congenital neutropenia due to other causes.[85,93] In two separate studies, iodine 125-SPA binding appeared more sensitive than the antiglobulin consumption assay or the functional opsonic assay for the detection of granulocyte antibodies.[90,94]

The failure of this technique to detect IgG3 and IgM antibodies is an important consideration. Verheugt and his associates determined the immunoglobulin class of 12 granulocyte-specific antibodies associated with alloimmune and autoimmune neutropenia, transfusion reactions, and polytransfused patients.[59] SPA would have failed to detect one IgM anti-NA1 antibody involved in a case of a febrile transfusion reaction, one IgG3 anti-NA2 antibody in a patient receiving granulocyte transfusions, and one case of autoimmune neutropenia due to an IgM and an IgA anti-ND1. Although granulocyte antibody was primarily associated with the presence of IgG1, six of the nine sera containing IgG1 activity also had IgG3 present, which shows the prevalence of that subclass with granulocyte antibody activity. In a report by McCullough et al,[29] SPA-detected antibodies in two children with autoimmune neutropenia did not correlate with the auto anti-NA1 detected by granulocyte agglutination or with the patients' neutropenic profiles.

Although the various findings do highlight the usefulness of this method for identifying granulocyte antibodies and studying granulocyte membrane alterations, they also underscore the limitations associated with the assay. It is suggested that the technique not be solely relied upon for the detection of all clinically significant granulocyte antibodies.

Avidin-Biotin Complex (ABC) Immunoassay There has recently been growing interest in the use of avidin- and biotin-conjugated reagents in immunoassays due to the high association constant of the glycoprotein avidin for the vitamin biotin ($K = 10^{-15}$ M) and its ability to conjugate proteins with many biotin groups per molecule without affecting activity contribute to this system's high sensitivity.[95]

There are three basic avidin-biotin techniques in common use: (1) labeled avidin-biotin (LAB),[96] (2) bridged avidin-biotin complex (BRAB),[96] and (3) avidin-biotin complex (ABC).[97,98] All three methods rely on the binding of biotinylated antibody to immobilized antigen, but differ in the specific method of label attachment.[99] The labels commonly used are fluorochromes such as fluorescein or rhodamine, enzymes such as peroxidase or alkaline phosphatase, or electron opaque-proteins such as ferritin.[99]

Using an avidin-biotin complex (ABC) immunoenzymatic system, Henke and his colleagues[100] developed an assay for visual detection of granulocyte surface antigens. A schematic diagram of the Henke's ABC test is depicted in Figure 2–6. Briefly, biotinylated anti-immunoglobulin bound to the primary antibody, is bridged by avidin to a biotinylated enzyme (horseradish peroxidase). An enzyme substrate, which allows the demonstration of antigen-antibody binding by an enzymatic reaction product, is then added. Advantages of the ABC system include good sensitivity which allows the study of heterogeneous cell populations and the reading of test results with light microscopy. It also successfully demonstrated the presence of HLA and granulocyte-specific antigens on the surface of granulocytes. The granulocytes were glutaraldehyde-fixed to slides and stored at $-80°C$ or $4°C$ for 1 week, thus eliminating the need for fresh cell preparations. However, it was noted that the antigenicity of cells stored at $4°C$ did decrease with time.

Enzyme-Linked Immunosorbent Assay (ELISA) First described by Engvall and Perlmann in 1971,[101] the assay has become very popular in providing the sensitivity associated with radioimmunoassays without the need for radioisotopes or expensive detection devices.[102] Briefly, immunoglobulin bound to the cell surface is detected by the addition of an enzyme conjugated to an antihuman immunoglobulin. The enzyme catalyzes a color change proportional to the antibody concentration when a specific substrate is added. Spectrophotometric measurement of the color provides quantitative analysis of the test reaction (Figure 2–7).

Utilization of the technique with platelet antibody testing has demonstrated the assay's sensitivity, specificity, reproducibility, and application for platelet compatibility testing and antibody identification.[103–105] Especially attractive for large-scale use was Schiffer and Young's[105] development of a micro ELISA system which uses

Figure 2–6.

Schematic representation of the avidin-biotin complex (ABC)
immunoenzymatic assay.

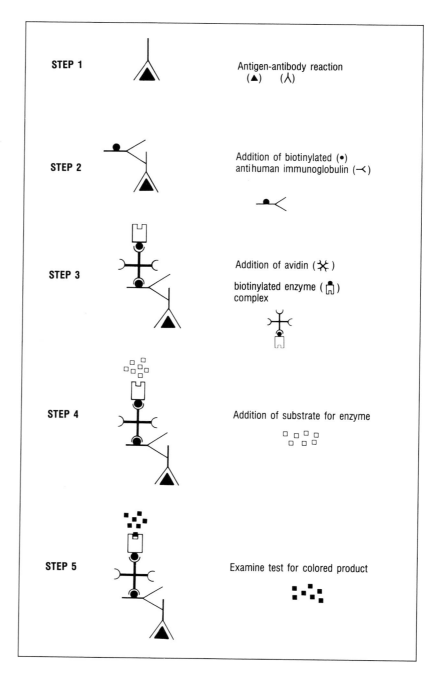

STEP 1 — Antigen-antibody reaction (▲) (人)

STEP 2 — Addition of biotinylated (•) antihuman immunoglobulin (—<)

STEP 3 — Addition of avidin (✕) biotinylated enzyme (⌂) complex

STEP 4 — Addition of substrate for enzyme

STEP 5 — Examine test for colored product

Figure 2–7.

Schematic representation of the granulocyte enzyme-linked immunosorbent assay (ELISA).

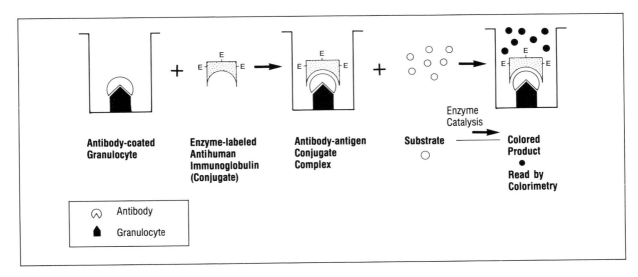

Antibody-coated Granulocyte + **Enzyme-labeled Antihuman Immunoglobulin (Conjugate)** → **Antibody-antigen Conjugate Complex** + **Substrate** → Enzyme Catalysis → **Colored Product Read by Colorimetry**

⌒ Antibody
▲ Granulocyte

microtiter plates, small reagent volumes, and cryopreserved dessicated cells.

Unfortunately, ELISA has not enjoyed similar success with granulocyte testing. The major problem involves finding a suitable conjugate-substrate reaction which will not be affected by the numerous intrinsic granulocyte enzymes. An alternative strategy would be attempting to use biochemical mechanisms to block or inactivate the intrinsic enzyme activity. Miller's group in St. Louis has not been successful in finding a suitable solution (Miller WV: personal communication), and Engelfriet's group,[60] after extensive testing, continued to have problems with nonspecific reactions that they were unable to resolve.

Recently, Mannoni and co-workers[106] described a granulocyte ELISA procedure used in their laboratory for screening monoclonal antibodies for myeloid and granulocyte specificity. Although the procedure appears encouraging, it remains to be seen whether it can be reproduced in other laboratories. The advantages of the assay and its potential for automation support efforts to adapt this technique for granulocyte serology.

Miscellaneous Binding Assays Felty's syndrome and systemic lupus erythematosus (SLE) patients' sera were examined for complement-fixing IgG granulocyte antibodies using a radiolabeled monoclonal anti-C3 in a direct binding assay.[94,107] Sera from seven of the 13 Felty's patients and ten of the 18 SLE patients studied found the 13 Felty's patients and ten of the 18 SLE patients studied found elevated amounts of C3, suggesting a role for complement-mediated injury in the pathophysiology of immune granulocytopenia. Cines et al[108] used a radiolabeled antiglobulin test to measure granulocyte-associated IgG in 16 patients with a variety of neutropenic disorders. Their study showed an inverse relationship between granulocyte-IgG levels and granulocyte counts, and suggested that a decrease of granulocyte-IgG was responsible for the steroid-induced clinical response in four patients treated with corticosteroids.

Antibody-Dependent Lymphocyte-Mediated Granulocyte Cytotoxicity (ADLG)

A fundamentally different approach to the detection of granulocyte antibodies utilizes killer cells (K-cells), a lymphocyte subpopulation capable of lysing antibody-sensitized target cells by antibody-dependent cell-mediated cytotoxicity. The acronym ADLG (antibody-dependent lymphocyte-mediated granulocyte cytotoxicity) was coined by Logue et al[109] when they applied the functional assay to the detection of antibodies bound to the surface of granulocytes. Prior to incubation with test serum, the target granulocytes are radiolabeled with chromium 51. The amount of chromium 51 released after lymphocyte-mediated (effector-mediated) cytolysis is measured with a gamma counter.

ADLG requires the interaction of Fc receptors (FcR) of K-cells with granulocyte-bound antibodies; therefore, K-cells must possess FcR for the class of bound antibody. Since both IgM and IgG induce K-cell–mediated ADLG, there are K-cells with IgG-FcR (FcγR), IgM-FcR (FcμR), or both. The precise lineage of the K-cell is still unknown. Presently, it appears that K-cell activity resides in T-cell and non-T, non-B cell (null) subsets of peripheral blood lymphocytes.[113] T-cells that function as K-cells in IgG-ADLG are referred to as Tγ cells. Proliferation of this cell subset in two patients with neutropenia and recurrent infections was reported by Bom-van Noorloos et al.[110] Recently, K-cells and T-cells have been categorized as subsets of an Fc receptor-bearing third population of human mononuclear cells with cytotoxic and regulatory function that have been called L cells.[111]

Cell lysis by K-cells is antibody-dependent and requires specific interaction of K-cell FcR with the Fc region of granulocyte-bound antibody (Figure 2–8). ADLG is not dependent on the complement system and is inhibited by cytochalasin-B. Aggregated IgG molecules, as in immune complexes, also interfere with reactions by binding firmly to lymphocyte FcR and blocking interaction with granulocyte-bound antibody.[112] The actual mechanism by which K-cells lyse antibody-sensitized granulocytes is not precisely known but has been presumed to be mediated via cytotoxic lymphokines.[113]

Figure 2–8.

Schematic representation of the antibody-dependent lymphocyte-mediated granulocyte cytotoxicity (ADLG) assay.

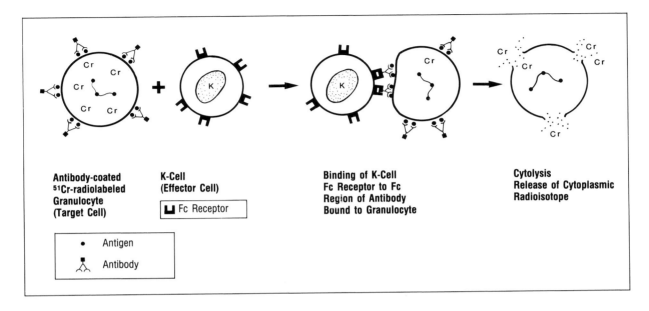

The pathogenetic role of granulocyte antibodies detected in the serum of patients with collagen vascular diseases, particulary Felty's syndrome and SLE, has been investigated by Logue and his associates using the ADLG assay.[109,114] Studies done in Engelfriet's laboratory have shown that both granulocyte-specific antibodies and HLA-specific antibodies can be detected by ADLG.[60] Antibody titration studies done in the same laboratory demonstrated that the ADLG assay is more sensitive than agglutination or immunofluorescence testing for detecting granulocyte-specific antibodies, and more sensitive than lymphocytotoxicity for HLA antibodies.[60] These observations suggest that the use of the assay for granulocyte antigen typing or identification of granulocyte antibody specificity would necessitate removal of contaminating HLA antibodies from the test serum. And, contrary to other findings, the Dutch investigators noted that immune complexes bound to the surface of granulocytes did not induce ADLG reactivity in their studies.[60]

Since ADLG assays may be subject to many technical variables, Richards et al[115] studied some of the possible contributing factors. ABO isohemagglutinins were shown to affect ADLG activity, thus requiring that appropriate controls be included when ABO-incompatible combinations are tested. ADLG activity was dependent on the source of effector cells and varied considerably among individuals. Storage of blood at room temperature for 24 hours and subsequent isolation of effector and target cells revealed loss of lymphocyte function, lower granulocyte-labeling efficiency, and higher granulocyte spontaneous chromium 51 release than fresh controls. Therefore, the choice of negative and positive control sera and strict attention to the technical aspects of this method are important.

As currently performed, the assay requires an effector cell: target cell ratio of 50:1, which results in the need for approximately 2×10^6 lymphocytes per test well. Variability of effector cell activity among donors necessitates standardization of the lymphocytes used in the test. The frequent need for large volumes of fresh lymphocytes from specified donors and the lengthy cell preparation procedure are major limitations to the use of this procedure for routine testing. Both factors could be addressed with the use of frozen lymphocytes obtained by lymphocyte apheresis. However, initial attempts in our laboratory to use cryopreserved effector cells obtained by phlebotomy have not been encouraging.

While the standard approach for antibody detection utilizes effector and corresponding autologous target cells from a cell donor, cells from other sources may be informative in ADLG testing. Lymphocytes and serum from an individual with a granulocyte antibody may be a more productive means of determining the in vivo effect of that antibody on donor cells. Furthermore, if sufficient granulocytes can be obtained from neutropenic patients for use as target cells, the assay may provide evidence for autologous mechanisms of in vivo granulocyte destruction in neutropenia.

Flow Cytofluorometry

Cells fluorescence-labeled by a variety of techniques can be subsequently analyzed by flow cytofluorometry, which provides quantitative measurement of single-cell fluorescence. By measuring both fluorescence intensity and light scatter, this technology permits evaluation of thousands of cells per second. Computer analysis of acquired data facilitates the detection and characterization of membrane antigen sites and subpopulations of cells. In addition to analyzing the cells, some flow cytometers are also cell sorters. These fluorescence-activated cell sorters (FACS) permit the selective isolation of subpopulations from a heterogeneous cell population.

With this instrumentation, fluorescence-tagged cells are channeled in a single file past a laser beam. Each cell passing through the laser beam produces two signals: the scatter signal, which is related to the size of the cell; and the fluorescence signal, which corresponds to the amount of bound antibody. Cell fluorescence measurements are recorded on a two-dimensional graph. The fluorescence intensity per cell is represented on the x axis as a series of channel units that range from low to high intensity. The number of cells per channel is recorded on the y axis. The analysis is displayed as a fluorescence distribution curve or histogram, and is often characterized by the peak channel of fluorescence and the mean channel of relative fluorescence. The peak channel is simply the channel in which the highest number of cells fluoresce. The mean channel is represented by the relative fluorescence intensity (RFI):[116]

$$\mathrm{RFI} = \frac{(\text{cells per channel} \times \text{channel-index number})}{\text{no. cells tested}}.$$

However, neither the mean cell channel nor the peak channel reflects the shape of the histogram. This shape often provides valuable information about the population analyzed. Several cell populations may display the same value of mean fluorescence intensity but have major differences in their distribution curves (Figure 2–9). Thus, it is important to evaluate the shape of the displayed data as well as the RFI.

Figure 2–9.

Illustration of fluorescence distribution displays for three different cell populations having the same mean peak channel of fluorescence intensity. (Adapted with permission from Patrick CW, Milson TJ, McFadden PW, Keller RH: Flow cytometry and cell sorting. Lab Med 15: 740–745, 1984).

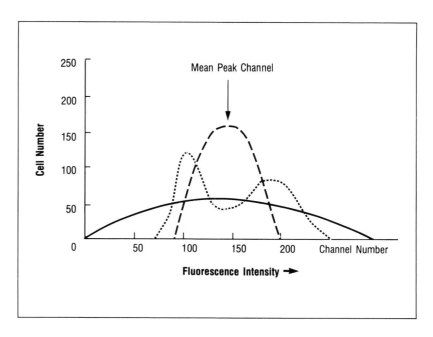

Granulocyte Functional Assays

Initially studied by Boxer and Stossel, a different approach to detecting granulocyte antibodies is based on their opsonic property and their ability to elicit or inhibit immune-mediated phagocytosis.[19,26] Other functional assays applied to the serologic study of immune neutropenia have included inhibition of myeloid maturation,[107,117,120] inhibition of neutrophil erythrophagocytosis,[118] and cell elastimetry measurements.[119] Although numerous investigations have been carried out using these techniques, their technical and serologic complexity together with their requirement for a large number of test cells and extensive time commitments, have diminished their practicality for routine or large-scale serologic testing.

Detection of Granulocyte-Associated Immunoglobulin

Most studies of immune granulocytopenia have focused on detecting circulating antibodies. This is largely due to the relative ease in obtaining serum from neutropenic patients versus the great difficulty in obtaining sufficient quantities of granulocytes for direct testing. Recently, however, it has been suggested that measurement of IgG on the granulocyte surface is more closely correlated with the presence of granulocytopenia.[108] Although 10 of the 12 patients studied had associated immunologic abnormalities and thus did not have primary autoimmune granulocytopenia, there was an inverse relationship between the amount of granulocyte-associated IgG and the granulocyte count. Patients with granulocytopenia secondary to intrinsic bone marrow disease, on myelosuppressive drugs, or with splenomegaly had normal levels of granulocyte-associated IgG. Four patients with increased granulocyte-associated IgG were treated with corticosteroids and experienced a decrease in the amount of granulocyte-associated IgG which correlated with an increase in granulocyte count. However, investigators employing other ways to measure granulocyte-associated IgG found no correlation between the quantity of granulocyte-associated IgG and the granulocyte count in patients with SLE[121] or Felty's syndrome.[122] Measurement of granulocyte-associated IgG has the potential to detect not only binding of autoantibodies but also coating of granulocytes with immune complexes containing IgG. Therefore, this may be a helpful approach in identifying patients with immune granulocytopenia.

Granulocyte Isolation From Neutropenic Patients

Unlike patients with hemolytic anemia, patients with severe neutropenia often do not have enough circulating granulocytes to isolate sufficient quantities for testing. In addition, it has been our experience that granulocytes from neutropenic patients demonstrate increased in vitro fragility and often do not separate normally on density separation gradients. Therefore, it may be difficult to obtain adequate numbers of cells for accurate analysis. The volume of blood required depends upon the patient's absolute neutrophil count. Our general guidelines are shown in Table 2–5.

Detection of in vivo cell-bound granulocyte antibodies is also challenging to the investigator due to intrinsic granulocyte properties. The high concentration of Fc receptors on granulocytes results in innate levels of cell-associated immunoglobulins and enhances the possibility for nonspecific binding of immune complexes or aggregated IgG complexes.[20,60,89] A further complication is associated with the granulocyte's capability of internalizing immunoglobulin bound to surface antigens. This process of antigenic modulation[89,123] was recently documented by Logue.[124] Furthermore, eluates prepared from an insufficient number of granulocytes are unreliable.[20]

Immunoglobulin Binding Assays

Most assays that detect granulocyte antibodies can be adapted to measure cell surface immunoglobulin in vivo. However, granulocyte agglutination and complement-dependent cytotoxicity that may be used for autologous serum-cell studies are not applicable for direct granulocyte antibody testing.

Quantitative assays that have been primarily employed for direct testing include antiglobulin consumption, Fab-anti-Fab, radiolabeled antiglobulin, SPA, and immunofluorescence. Recent interest has focused on the last three, with immunofluorescence currently being the most widely used serologic technique, primarily because of its ability to detect all immunoglobulin classes. The major difficulty in using the GIF assay to detect cell-bound IgG is in distinguishing between immune complexes and cell-bound antibodies. Approaches to solving this problem are discussed in chapter 4, Immune Complexes. As in vitro immunoglobulin binding increases

Table 2–5.	Volume of Blood Required for Direct Antibody Testing or Granulocyte Typing

Absolute Neutrophil Count/μL	Required Blood Volume (mL)
>2000	20
1500–2000	30–40
1000–1500	50
<1000	*

* Obtaining sufficient granulocytes for testing at this level is difficult.

with time and granulocytes are kept in whole blood storage prior to isolation and testing, this must also be considered. We tested granulocytes from normal panel donors in the GIF assay after incubation of whole blood prior to isolation for 24 hours at 4°C, 22°C, and 37°C. The direct fluorescence of these stored cells was always greater than that of cells from the same donors processed within 2 hours of collection.

SPA only reacts with the Fc region of surface-bound immunoglobulin, the steric presentation considered to be associated with immune-mediated granulocyte destruction.[89] This specificity gives the SPA assay an advantage not present with fluorescent- or radioactively-tagged immunoglobulin conjugates.

The slide SPA technique in which washed blood films from patients can be directly analyzed has the additional advantage of obtaining adequate quantities of cells from neutropenic patients. However, current experience with this method for such testing is limited.

Although direct quantitation of granulocyte-bound IgG is possible with the iodine 125 anti-IgG binding test developed by Cines et al,[108] the difficulty in performing thorough testing on insufficient quantities of cells from neutropenic patients was noted. This problem can be addressed by the use of flow cytofluorometry, which can produce accurate results on low counts with a heterogeneous cell population. When using a fluorescence intensity index to measure granulocyte fluorescence, relative amounts of autoantibody can be semiquantitated and followed during the course of the patient's autoimmune neutropenia.

Identification of Immunoproteins Bound In Vivo

Immunoglobulin Class   The ability to determine the specific immunoglobulin class of antibody bound in vivo is currently limited to the following techniques: (1) fluorescein isothiocyanate (FITC)- or tetramethylrhodamine isothiocyanate (TRITC)-labeled antihuman immunoglobulins (anti-IgG, anti-IgM, anti-IgA) with the GIF assay, and (2) biotinylated antihuman immunoglobulin (IgG, IgM, IgA) with the avidin-biotin immunoenzymatic assay. Antibody detected by the SPA and radiolabeled antiglobulin binding assay is primarily IgG.

Since the publication by Verheugt's group in 1978[59] describing the IgG subclass composition of granulocyte alloantibodies and autoantibodies, there has been much interest among granulocyte serologists in having available subclass antisera for continued studies of this nature. FITC-labeled IgG subclass-specific antisera can be obtained commercially (Central Laboratory of the Netherlands Red Cross Blood Transfusion Service, or Accurate Chemical and Scientific Corp., Westbury, NY) but are not available as $F(ab')_2$ fragments. This, and the problems of obtaining controls, make interpretation difficult.

Complement Components Direct examination of granulocytes from neutropenic patients for in vivo complement deposition has primarily been done with the SPA slide test. This uses a suspension of protein A containing staphylococci and rabbit antihuman complement serum (anti-C3b, -C3d, and -C4). With this procedure, Harmon et al[90] tested the neutrophils from 35 neutropenic individuals and found three that had granulocyte-associated complement without IgG. FITC- and iodine 125-labeled anti-C3 reagents have also been successfully used with the GIF assay and a surface binding assay, respectively, to determine the C3-fixing capacity of granulocyte antibodies found in patient serum samples,[59,94,107] but little information is available on their use in direct testing. However, an attempt by Minchinton's group[125] to use FITC-labeled anti-C3 for granulocyte antibody investigations in bone marrow transplant recipients was unsuccessful due to the high background fluorescence associated with the anti-C3 reagent used.

Chapter 3

Other Granulocyte Serologic Techniques

Granulocyte Preservation

The fundamental problem associated with the development and application of granulocyte antibody testing is the need to obtain viable, functionally intact granulocytes. A few assays that use cells preserved for up to 3 weeks are beginning to emerge, but they have not yet been extensively evaluated.[90] There is a substantial need for a procedure for long-term preservation of cells for use in a variety of assays. Thus, we investigated the use of frozen granulocytes and granulocyte cytoplasts in the GA and GIF assays.

Frozen Granulocytes

Much effort has been directed toward freezing granulocytes for transfusion. Although the results reported vary among investigators, most studies have shown a progressive loss of granulocyte viability and function upon freezing and thawing.[126-130] However, the use of frozen granulocytes for serologic testing has not yet been established. Using a modification of Richman's freezing protocol,[126] in which granulocytes suspended in phosphate buffer are frozen in 10% DMSO at $-80°C$, we compared GA and GIF granulocyte antigen typings of frozen and fresh granulocytes from six normal donors. The granulocytes were nonreactive in the GA assay. This result appeared to be related to loss of cell viability. For use in the GIF assay, the granulocytes were treated with PFA either before or after freezing. The average postthaw recovery of the unfixed cells was 65% versus 84% for PFA-fixed cells. The cells were difficult to read, and membrane damage was apparent from the number of cells with cytoplasmic fluorescence. The following criteria were used for interpretation of results: (1) 0% to 50%

damaged cells were interpretable, (2) 50% to 90% damaged cells were difficult to interpret, and (3) 90% to 100% damaged cells were not interpretable. Of the 61 typing reactions analyzed using cells frozen before PFA treatment, 45 (74%) were difficult to interpret and 16 (26%) could not be evaluated. With the PFA-fixed cells, 28 (46%) of the tests were interpretable, 24 (39%) of the tests were difficult to interpret, and 9 (15%) were not interpretable. Both frozen cell preparations demonstrated acceptable levels of accuracy (85%) and sensitivity (94%) compared with fresh granulocyte antigen typing, but the high (35%) rate of false positive reactions would be a major impediment to using frozen granulocytes in this assay.

Thus, our studies suggest that (1) frozen granulocytes do not appear suitable for GA testing, (2) PFA treatment of granulocytes prior to freezing was associated with increased cell recoveries and decreased cell damage, and (3) frozen PFA-treated granulocytes may have limited applications in GIF testing. However, damaged cells make interpretations difficult or, in some cases, impossible. Due to the substantial nonspecific binding reflected by the high false positive rate, weakly reactive antibodies may be difficult to detect using frozen granulocytes.

Granulocyte Cytoplasts (Neutroplasts)

The production of enucleated granulocytes by Roos and his associates in 1983[131] and subsequent successful cryopreservation of these cells by Voetman et al[132] introduced an exciting new approach to the study of granulocyte membrane structures or functions without the problems previously associated with nuclear or cytoplasmic granule interactions. For granulocyte serologists, van der Veen's[133] application of both fresh and frozen granulocyte cytoplasts (neutroplasts) to granulocyte antibody testing using GA and GIF was a major advance in the development and growth of granulocyte immunology. Although this is not a simple procedure, the production of neutroplasts can be performed by most laboratories and takes about 4 hours, as outlined in Figure 3–1.

To investigate the potential use of cytoplasts in our serology program, we have done a few preliminary studies comparing GA and GIF reactivity of fresh neutroplasts to fresh granulocytes using selected granulocyte antibodies. On one occasion, granulocytes and neutroplasts from the same donor were typed for NA1, NA2, NB1, and NB2 antigens using the GA assay. The granulocytes typed positive for all four antigens, but no reactivity was noted with the neutroplasts. This is consistent with their known lack of motility. We did not employ van der Veen's modification of the GA assay that allowed use of neutroplasts in that test system.[133] When selected dilutions of NA1, NA2, and NB1 antibodies were tested with cell preparations from three donors using the GIF assay, antibody titers with neutroplasts were lower than with granulocytes in four

Figure 3–1.

Flow diagram depicting the major steps in the preparation and isolation of neutroplasts from whole blood.

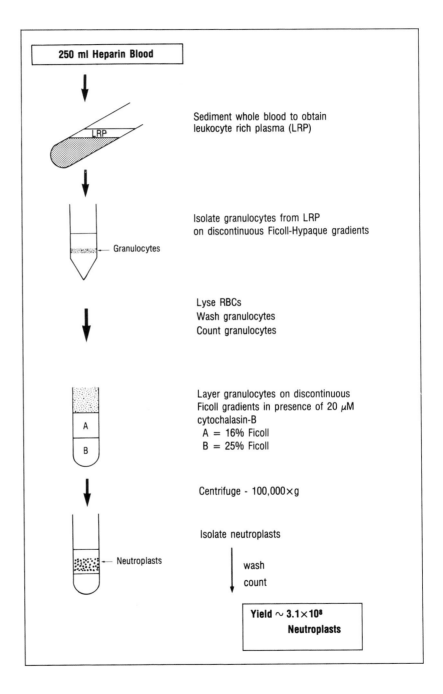

Table 3–1.

Reactivity of Fresh Granulocytes (PMN) and Neutroplasts (PLAST)

	Donor Typing				Antibodies								
	Granulocyte[a]			HLA[b]	Granulocyte							HLA	
					NA1		NA2		NB1			B7	
No.	NA1	NA2	NB1	B7	PMN	PLAST	PMN	PLAST	PMN	PLAST		PMN	PLAST
1	−	+	+	NT	0	0	1000	100	100	100		NT	NT
2	−	+	−	NT	0	0	500	50	1000	100		NT	NT
3	+	−	+	+	500	50	0	0	500	500		+[c]	+[c]

NOTE: Antibodies were tested in GIF at dilutions of 1:10, 1:50, 1:100, 1:500, 1:1000; and the last reciprocal of the dilution giving a positive reaction was noted.
[a] Determined by granulocyte agglutination.
[b] Determined by lymphocytotoxicity.
[c] Titers not done — 4+ reaction at 1:15 antibody dilution.
ABBREVIATION: NT = not tested.

Table 3–2.

Neutroplast and Granulocyte Antigen Typing Reactions

		Neutroplast	
		+	−
Granulocyte	+	26	8
	−	0	18
		$p < .001$ (χ^2)	

NOTE: Reagents used: Anti-NA1, anti-NA2, anti-NB1, negative and positive control sera. Assay used: GIF.

of the six positive typing reactions (Table 3–1). Donor 2 typed as NB1 negative in the GA assay, but typed positive with GIF. We have now seen this discrepancy with other GA NB1-negative individuals. Donor 3 was HLA-B7 positive and anti-B7 reacted with both cell preparations, demonstrating the retention of HLA antigens on neutroplasts.

Granulocytes and neutroplasts from ten normal donors were tested with selected granulocyte antibodies and evaluated by GIF (Table 3–2). Although there was a significant correlation ($p < .001$) of reactions between both cell preparations, the incidence of false negative results with neutroplasts was 23%, which resulted in an overall accuracy of 85%. Again, this reflects the weaker reactivity of neutroplasts, which suggests that some amount of membrane antigen has been removed or modified during the enucleation procedure. Van der Veen also noticed a slight decrease in granulocyte antibody titer with neutroplasts.[133]

Much is yet to be learned about this new granulocyte product, but it is clear that neutroplasts can be used for GIF testing. Technical advances will, hopefully, improve sensitivity. Due to the contribution of the Dutch scientists, the possibility for preserved cell panels and exchange of cells among laboratories now truly exists.

Elution of Granulocyte Antibodies

In their identification of the first granulocyte-specific antigen (NA1), Lalezari et al[11] used heat (56°C) for the elution of antibodies from sensitized granulocytes to demonstrate their neutrophil specificity. Helmerhorst et al[134] later compared four different elution methods (low pH, DMSO, ether, and 56°C heat) for removal of alloantibodies and autoantibodies from sensitized granulocytes. Granulocyte antibodies were best eluted by lowering the pH of the medium. In their study, only NA2 antibodies were eluted by all four methods. Other granulocyte-specific and HLA antibodies demonstrated activity only after low pH elution. Antibody titers were lower in the eluates than in the original serum, and antibodies reactive only by GA were negative or much weaker in the eluates than antibodies detected by the GIF test.[134] Unfortunately, the method as it is currently performed[20,134] is technically involved, requires numerous granulocytes and takes 1 day to perform, making it impractical for routine use.

Methods for Eliminating Human Leukocyte Antigen (HLA) Reactivity

Platelet Absorption

Because of the large number of stable HLA antigens on platelets and utilization of outdated platelet concentrates as a source of absorbing cells, this procedure has been widely used for the removal of HLA-A, HLA-B, and HLA-C antibodies for both lymphocyte and granulocyte serologic testing procedures. Postabsorption serum must be retested for HLA activity to confirm complete absorption of HLA antibodies. During the absorption procedure, platelet fragments, which make interpretation of some assays difficult, may be introduced. These may be removed by centrifugation. Although platelets do not contain granulocyte-specific antigens, we have observed loss of reactivity of some weakly reactive granulocyte-specific antibodies following platelet absorption, possibly due to manipulation or inadvertent dilution.

Chloroquine Stripping

Chloroquine, an antimalarial drug known to dissociate immune complexes and remove antibody from red blood cell surfaces,[135] has been shown by Blumberg et al to be effective in removing HLA-A and HLA-B antigens from platelets.[136] Evidence that this antigen stripping procedure eliminated HLA antibody reactions while not affecting platelet-specific antibody-antigen reactivity was provided by Nordhagen and Flaathen.[137] Recently, the use of chloroquine to remove HLA antigens from granulocytes without removal of granulocyte-specific antigens was introduced by Minchinton and Waters.[138] They reported the removal of HLA antigens A1, A2, A3, B7, B8, B27, and B40 from chloroquine-treated granulocytes with no loss of NA1 or NA2 antigen activity as compared to nontreated cells. Initial trials of this new technique in our laboratory were unsuccessful but suggested that the commercial source or the preparation of chloroquine used may be critical. Further studies need to be done to establish this intriguing approach to the elimination of HLA antibody contamination in granulocyte serology testing.

Detection of Drug-Related Antibodies

Both toxic and immunologic mechanisms have been associated with drug-related agranulocytosis, and numerous drugs have been implicated.[139] Although the serologic techniques for the detection of drug-associated granulocyte antibodies are not well developed or standardized, certain assays have successfully demonstrated the presence of drug antibodies. As the drug must usually be present in the in vitro tests for antibody detection, two mechanisms similar to those observed in certain drug-induced hemolytic anemias are suggested for the drug-induced immunologic granulocyte damage:[140] (1) formation of drug-dependent immune complexes that bind to the granulocyte membrane (eg, quinidine), and (2) attachment of the drug to the cell surface where it functions as a hapten and elicits antibody formation (eg, penicillin). However, in some in vitro studies the drug was not necessary or did not potentiate the reactions, and antibody activity was present long after cessation of drug therapy.[140,141] This suggests drug induction of granulocyte autoantibodies that react with the cells.

Drug-related granulocyte agglutinating antibodies have been detected in association with aminopyrine, sulfonamides, quinidine, antithyroid drugs, cephradine, and B-lactamine.[6,142-146] Opsonizing drug-associated granulocyte antibodies were demonstrated in the sera of 16 patients suspected of having drug-induced neutropenia. The drugs involved were synthetic penicillins (nafcillin, dicloxacillin, oxacillin), procainamide, sulfafurazole, cephalothin, vancomycin, propylthiouracil, methimazole, gold thiomalate, and quinidine.[140,147,148] Opsonic antibody activity independent of complement, but dependent on drug concentrations, was demonstrated in the patients receiving synthetic penicillin, whereas complement-dependent IgM opsonic antibody was detected in the patient receiving methimazole.[140] Specific IgM granulocytotoxic, drug-independent autoantibodies associated with granulocytopenia have been demonstrated in patients receiving levaminsole, propylthiouracil, and aprindine.[141,149-151] The immunofluorescence assay has been used for the study of quinine- and quinidine-associated thrombocytopenia[152] and can similarly be applied to granulocytopenia drug studies. Recently, the ADLG assay was used to reveal a cell-mediated immune mechanism associated with procainamide-induced agranulocytosis.[153]

Studies of the kinetics of these drug-associated antibodies have shown that although the initial antibody titer or strength of reactivity may be high, antibody activity quickly declines after discontinuation of the drug and is usually absent upon return of normal granulocyte counts.[140,141,146,149-151] This was especially emphasized in the study of patients with neutropenia due to B-lactamine antibodies.[146] The antibody titers were low, and in one case, antibody activity was gone 5 days after discontinuation of the drug. In this study, serum was obtained within 1 day after the drug was stopped and did not require the addition of drug to demonstrate drug antibody activity. However, when using serum from day 2 or 3, agglutination was more easily detected with drug addition.

Hence, for successful detection of drug-induced granulocyte antibodies, it is important to obtain patient serum samples during the nadir of the granulocytopenia, soon after the drug has been discontinued and after the patient's granulocyte count has returned to normal. If these sera fail to react with a panel of donor granulocytes, conclusive evidence for the presence of a drug-associated autoimmune mechanism may be obtained by testing the patient's granulocytes upon recovery with the patient's serum (with and without the addition of drug) obtained during various phases of the disease course.

Detection of Cold-Reacting Antibodies

First described by Lalezari and Murphy[154] in 1967, cold-reacting granulocyte antibodies initially appeared to be related to the presence of I-i determinants on granulocytes, but several examples that demonstrated no corresponding red blood cell antigen specificity were found. A few reports have suggested that these antibodies may be pathogenically related to the neutropenias associated with certain cases of infectious mononucleosis, Mycoplasma pneumonia, or severe chronic neutropenia.[57,63,154,155] Lalezari has subsequently reported that approximately 25% of normal individuals have "naturally occurring" cold granulocyte agglutinins with titers not exceeding 8, whereas pathologic cold GA antibody titers are greater than 16.[56]

Cold-reacting granulocyte antibodies have been detected primarily with the GA and the GIF assays, but other assays can be modified with precooled reagents, 4°C serum-cell incubation, and rapid evaluation of test results to minimize exposure to warm conditions during analysis. For the GIF technique, Lalezari[56] recommends that FITC-labeled anti-IgM and anti-IgG should be incubated with the sensitized cells for 30 minutes at 4°C and 30 minutes at 18°C.

Determination of Monospecificity of Unknown Antibodies

A previously unrecognized antibody may in fact be defining multiple specificities rather than a single antigen. This is especially important to consider with apparent high-frequency antibodies. Although time consuming, one method to exclude this possibility involves absorption of the serum with separate aliquots of granulocytes from ten different donors (See Granulocyte Absorption Method, procedure 3.2A). Each of the absorbed aliquots is then tested with a panel of cells. If the antibody is reacting with a single high-incidence antigen, cell activity will have been removed by each absorption. However, in a serum containing a mixture of antibodies, the chances are that some absorptions will only partially remove reactivity, depending upon which antigens are expressed by the absorbing cell. When tested against the cell panel, absorbed aliquots will give varying results.

Testing for Soluble Antigens

It is useful to know whether an antigen being investigated occurs in a soluble form in plasma. As antigens present in a soluble form in body fluids are well characterized, this information might aid in determining the nature and specificity of the antigen being investigated. Plasma from two donors—one whose cells are reactive and one whose cells are nonreactive with the antibody being investigated—is used. The serum containing the antibody is titrated, using plasma from each donor as a diluent, and the results are compared. If the plasma from the reactive donor reduces the titer compared with plasma from the nonreactive donor, then it is likely that the antigen does occur in plasma and further investigation is warranted.

Preservation of Granulocyte Antibodies

A collection of granulocyte antisera is one of the most valuable assets of a granulocyte antibody laboratory. Accurate granulocyte typing of patients or panel donors requires use of more than one antiserum for any given known specificity due to variability of antigen expression, antibody strength, and possible contaminating nonspecific reactivity. It is also important to have a battery of sera from patients known to have immune-mediated granulocytopenias in evaluating new tests for their suitability for the detection of granulocyte antibodies. Because of the extreme value of these sera, they should be handled and preserved with extraordinary care.

We believe that the following guidelines are important in developing and maintaining a collection of sera containing granulocyte antibodies:

1. Develop a classification and labeling system permitting stored samples to be easily located. Records containing serologic testing results, as well as clinical and laboratory data of the serum donor, must also be readily accessible.

2. Store samples as serum whenever possible. We have found that plasma should be promptly recalcified before freezing. Poor clot formation may occur with postfreezing recalcification. This results in fibrin clots, which may make the interpretation of certain assays difficult, if not impossible.

3. Store serum samples at the lowest available freezer temperatures, but never above $-20°C$.

4. Use durable plastic freezer vials that can be easily and permanently labeled with the information necessary to identify the sample.

5. Store samples in small aliquots to avoid repeated thawing and freezing, which may often cause antibody deterioration.

6. Optimally, sera should be shipped frozen in sufficient dry ice (5 lb minimum), and delivered within 24 hours. Although we have detected antibodies in sera shipped at uncontrolled temperatures, loss of antibody reactivity cannot be excluded when negative results occur in such sera. A major problem associated with sera remaining at warm temperatures for an extended period is the risk of bacterial contamination, which then renders the sample unsuitable for testing.

7. Sera may be heat-inactivated before or after freezing. We heated eight sera, including antibodies to NA1 and NA2, to $56°C$ for 30 minutes. We then assayed their activity by both titration endpoints and by titration scores and found no significant difference in antibody reactivity between heated and unheated sera in either granulocyte immunofluorescence or granulocyte agglutination.

Chapter 4

Interfering Factors in Granulocyte Antibody Assays

Anti-A, Anti-B, Anti-A,B

Controversy associated with the expression of ABH antigen on granulocytes has historically dictated the use of ABO compatible granulocytes for antibody screening and AB sera for negative control reagents (see chapter 6). There is no direct evidence that anti-A, anti-B, or anti-A,B are reactive with granulocytes in either the GA or the GIF assay.[20,81,156] Isohemagglutinins were shown by Richards et al[115] to have an effect in the ADLG assay, but had no effect in the same assay in a study done by van der Veen.[133] The discrepancy between these two observations may have involved the quantity of red blood cells in the granulocyte preparations used in their studies; Richards used discontinuous Ficoll-Hypaque–prepared granulocytes without hypotonic lysis, whereas van der Veen employed red blood cell hypotonic lysis in his cell preparation. We have found that Ficoll-Hypaque–isolated granulocytes can have an average of 8% red blood cells (Table 2–2).

Since the issue is still unresolved, the current standard granulocyte procedure is to continue the use of ABO-compatible testing situations whenever feasible. Acceptance of recent evidence indicating the lack of ABH antigen expression on granulocytes[157–161] may change standard practices.

Human Leukocyte Antigen (HLA) Antibodies

HLA-A and HLA-B antigens have been shown to be on the surface of granulocytes,[57,64,162] although with lower density than on lymphocytes, and are variably expressed.[163] The detection of HLA antibodies in the GA, GIF, and ADLG assays has been well documented.[60,81,164] Thus, HLA antibodies can potentially interfere in the serologic detection or characterization of granulocyte-specific antibodies. Contamination of granulocyte typing sera with HLA antibodies can also cause false positive reactions. For these reasons, it is often desirable to differentiate HLA antibodies from granulocyte-specific antibodies. Two approaches are currently available to remove contaminating HLA reactivity: (1) platelet absorption of test serum, and (2) chloroquine stripping of HLA antigens from granulocytes (see chapter 3).

Immune Complexes

Immune complexes are capable of binding to granulocyte membranes through interaction with granulocyte Fc receptors for IgG or complement receptors CR1 and CR3.[60] Their interference in granulocyte antibody assays is variable. The contribution of immune complexes to the levels of granulocyte-associated IgG in SLE and Felty's patients has been primarily studied with the Fab anti-Fab assay.[121,165] Sera containing immune complexes from nonneutropenic patients did not sensitize granulocytes as detected by binding of SPA.[60] Large IgG aggregates caused positive reactions in the GA assays, but immune complexes did not.[60] Immune complexes did not induce complement-dependent or lymphocyte-mediated granulocytotoxicity.[60,78] Both immune complexes formed in vitro (tetanus/antitetanus and DNA/anti-DNA), and aggregated IgG gave positive reactions in the GIF assay.[60] Since both granulocyte antibodies and immune complexes are detected by the GIF assay, it is sometimes necessary to try to distinguish which may be involved in a positive test reaction. The following approaches may be used:[60] (1) the patient's serum can be tested for the presence of immune complexes using standard techniques such as an iodine 125-C1q binding assay, (2) an eluate can be prepared and tested for specificity, and (3) granulocyte FcR monoclonal antibodies can be used to inhibit antibody binding in the presence of immune complexes.

If reactivity with the eluate or serum demonstrates a granulocyte specificity or a polymorphic profile, it is most likely that an antibody is present. Conversely, if the eluate lacks any reactivity or no polymorphism can be detected, it is more suggestive of the presence of immune complex reactivity. Because of the technical problems with granulocyte elution, preliminary results from Engelfriet's group using the FcR monoclonal antibody approach are most encouraging. First, they demonstrated that when granulocyte FcR are blocked by monoclonal antibodies, the FcR of granulocytes did not adhere to IgG-coated red blood cells. Second, when these same granulocytes were analyzed in the GIF assay, the FcR monoclonal antibody reduced or eliminated the binding of aggregated IgG, but did not interfere with the binding of a granulocyte-specific antibody (anti-NA1).[60]

Immune complexes have been reported in a high proportion of patients with chronic idiopathic granulocytopenia.[166,167] Sera from

43 patients with autoimmune disease associated with circulating immune complexes demonstrated a significant correlation between GIF and C1q-binding activity.[60] To investigate the potential involvement of immune complexes in juvenile autoimmune neutropenia (AIN), we examined their correlation with granulocyte antibodies detected in this patient group. Sera from 29 juvenile patients with primary AIN were tested for granulocyte antibodies using the GA and GIF assays and for immune complexes with an iodine 125-C1q binding test. Although all the patients had GA and/or GIF antibodies, only two had immune complexes detected in their sera (Table 4–1). Sixteen of the 29 antibodies were specific for known granulocyte antigens (15 NA1, 1 NA2), but those were not associated with the presence of immune complexes. Thus, our studies do not indicate a significant involvement of immune complexes in juvenile AIN.

Table 4–1.   ***Correlation of Immune Complexes with Granulocyte Antibodies in 29 Patients with Juvenile Primary Autoimmune Neutropenia***

		Granulocyte Antibodies			
		GA		GIF	
		+	−	+	−
Immune	+	2	0	2	0
Complexes*	−	27	0	26	1

* Determined by iodine 125-C1q binding assay.

Chapter 5

Characterization of Granulocyte Antibodies

Limited information is available regarding the immunochemical and serologic properties of granulocyte-specific antibodies. However, additional studies relating the immunochemical nature of granulocyte antibodies to their serologic reactivities and in vivo effects would be useful in designing and selecting assays for the clinical application of granulocyte serology.

Immunochemical Characteristics

The most extensive investigation of the immunochemical properties of granulocyte antibodies was performed by Verheugt and his associates.[59] Using the GIF assay, they determined the immunoglobulin class, subclass, and light-chain composition of 12 granulocyte-specific antibodies from five patients with alloimmune neonatal neutropenia, three patients with autoimmune neutropenia, two patients with febrile transfusion reactions, one patient who received massive platelet transfusions, and one patient receiving granulocyte transfusions. Ten of the 12 antibodies were IgG. One of the two patients experiencing febrile transfusion reactions had an IgM antibody with NA1 specificity, and one autoantibody with ND1 specificity was shown to consist of IgM and IgA. IgG antibody subclass examinations revealed that three specimens were IgG1, one was IgG3, five were composed of IgG1 and IgG3 antibodies, and one patient had IgG1, IgG2, IgG3, and IgG4 antibodies present. No relationship between the immunoglobulin class or IgG subclass and the clinical effect of the granulocyte-specific antibodies was seen. Six of the nine antibodies tested had both k and λ light chain composition, while three demonstrated only λ light chains.

We recently determined the immunoglobulin class of GIF antibodies from 27 juvenile patients with primary autoimmune neutropenia using class-specific fluoresceinated antibody conjugates. Nineteen patients had only IgG antibody, two patients had only IgM antibody, five patients had IgG and IgM antibody activity, and in one patient IgM and IgA antibodies were present. Fifteen of the 27 antibodies had anti-NA1 specificity that was primarily IgG, although IgM activity was detected. (NA1 specificity was detected in 11 of the 19 IgG antibodies and in 4 of the 5 IgG + IgM antibody combinations.)

Clinically significant granulocyte antibodies appear to be predominantly IgG. However, IgM and IgA antibodies occur with some frequency, indicating the necessity for inclusion of assays capable of their detection in screening protocols.

Serological Characteristics

Granulocyte agglutinins are usually IgG, although IgM and mixtures of IgG, IgM, and IgA have been reported[59] and observed in our laboratory. Granulocyte cytotoxins are usually IgM,[59,78,79,140,150] but may occasionally be IgG.[59,76,77] Fractionation of sera from patients with autoimmune neutropenia reactive in ADLG revealed the active component to be contained in the IgG-containing fraction.[108] Verheugt's study showed that the immunochemical properties of granulocyte antibodies correlated strongly with their serological behavior.[59] IgG granulocyte agglutinins had optimum reactivity at 37°C, while IgM agglutinins and cytotoxins were best detected at 22°C or lower temperatures. In the GIF assay no significant difference in the amount of IgG antibody binding was found using 4°C, 22°C, or 37°C incubations, nor was there any correlation between the IgG subclass composition of the IgG antibodies and their reactivity at different temperatures. One of two IgM antibodies studied had enhanced binding at 4°C and equivocal binding at 22°C and 37°C. The IgM granulocyte alloantibody, but not the IgM autoantibody, demonstrated complement binding in the GC and anticomplement fluorescence technique. This suggests that non–complement binding IgM antibodies do occur. In addition, reactivity of IgG antibodies in the GC and anticomplement fluorescence assay suggested that some IgG antibodies are capable of complement binding. This observation has been confirmed by Rustagi et al.[168]

It has been reported that IgG antibodies produce round agglutinates, whereas IgM antibodies produced agglutinates with a looser and more irregular shape.[59] We were unable to confirm this observation when we tested granulocytes from a donor positive for both the NA1 and NB1 antigen with three antibodies in the GA assay: (1) IgM anti-NA1, (2) IgG anti-NA1, and (3) IgG anti-NB1. The antibodies were serially diluted, incubated for 4 hours at 30°C with the test granulocytes, and subsequently examined at a selected dilution for comparison of agglutinate appearance. As shown in Figures 5–1A through D, both IgG and IgM antibodies produced round agglutinates, and the looser appearing agglutination occurred with the IgG anti-NB1 antibody. Therefore, the appearance of the agglutinates in the GA assay does not necessarily correlate with antibody immunoglobulin class.

Autoantibodies Versus Alloantibodies

A phenomenon regularly noted in the serologic investigation of warm autoimmune hemolytic anemia is that of an antibody eluate

Figure 5–1.

Appearance of agglutinates of NA1- and NB1-positive granulocytes after 4 hours incubation with IgG and IgM antibodies (diluted 1:4) in the GA assay. (A) Tight agglutinates formed with an IgG anti-NA1, (B) loose agglutinates formed with an IgG anti-NB1, (C) small tight agglutinates formed with an IgM anti-NA1, (D) negative control.

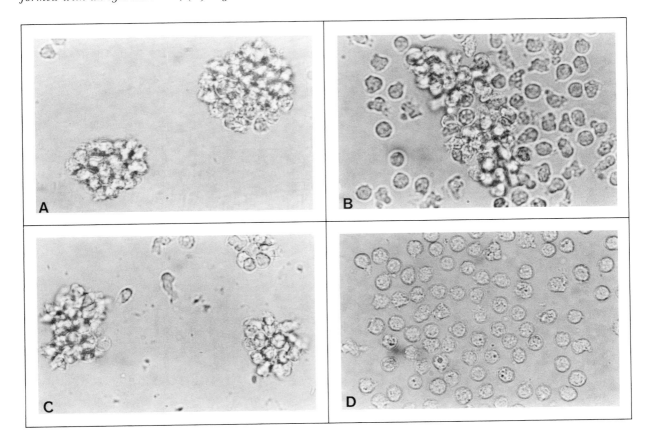

showing an apparent blood group specificity for an antigen that was not detected on the patient's red blood cells,[169] eg, anti-E eluted from E-negative red blood cells. In a study of 48 autoantibodies with simple Rh specificities, Issitt[170] showed that 34 (71%) of these autoantibodies could be absorbed by red blood cells that lacked the corresponding antigens. Autoantibodies such as these (so-called mimicking autoantibodies) were obviously fundamentally different from alloantibodies of corresponding specificities which cannot be absorbed by cells that lack the appropriate antigens.

Several of the reported granulocyte-specific antigens have been characterized on the basis of autoantibodies from patients with autoimmune neutropenia. Because of the above observations, we examined some of the granulocyte autoantibodies previously studied in our laboratory for occurrence of a similar phenomenon. We absorbed four examples of autoanti-NA1 with granulocytes expressing and granulocytes lacking NA1. One NA1 autoantibody was completely absorbed with granulocytes that were either NA1-positive or NA1-negative. The other three sera lost anti-NA1 activity only when the absorbing cell expressed the NA1 antigen. Although these preliminary findings must be confirmed with additional absorptions with other examples of autoantibodies, one autoantibody was absorbed with cells that apparently lack the appropriate antigen. This suggests that a similar phenomenon to red blood cell mimicking autoantibodies may also occur with granulocyte autoantibodies.

It also may be important, when performing serologic or immunogenetic studies with granulocyte autoantibodies, to bear in mind that the specificities may be different than with corresponding alloantibodies. For example, we have found several autoantibodies which reacted with all donor granulocytes, showing specificity only when titrated. Alloantibodies, when free of HLA contamination, demonstrate specificity more readily with little or no dilution.

Chapter 6

Granulocyte Antigens

Cell surface alloantigens found on granulocytes fall into two major categories and several subcategories, based upon their distribution on various cell lines.[57,60,157,171–172] The major categories are (1) tissue-specific antigens, which are found exclusively on cells of a particular lineage or cells that arise from common precursors; and (2) systemic antigens, which are distributed on several apparently ontogenetically unrelated cell lines. As Lalezari pointed out,[157] the major groups into which antigens fall, in addition to the pattern of antigenic change observed in maturing cells, may provide important clues to the biological role of these antigens.

Some of the major difficulties of working with the granulocyte-specific antigens include the problems that are inherent in the techniques for detecting antibodies directed against granulocyte antigens. These difficulties are a result of the numerous methods used to define antigens, the apparent lack of correlation among the results obtained with these different assays, and the fact that virtually all of these techniques require the testing of fresh samples of granulocytes. Since many of these antigens are of relatively high incidence, it is usually very difficult to obtain cells lacking the antigens. The requirement for fresh granulocytes makes comparisons of reactions with rare cells among different laboratories almost impossible due to problems with shipping conditions and testing delays. An additional problem involves the short supply of many of the sera that define granulocyte antigens, precluding exchange among laboratories.

A major advance in the field of granulocyte serology would be the organization of a workshop or program of sera exchange, permitting the systematic comparison and investigation of the multitude of antigens described in different laboratories. In addition, the cell line distribution of many of these antigens could be more completely characterized.

Tissue-Specific Antigens

Tissue-specific alloantigens detected on granulocytes may be divided into two main categories: (1) granulocyte-specific antigens, and (2) granulocyte-monocyte antigens.

Granulocyte-Specific Antigens

Granulocyte-specific antigens are those with tissue distribution restricted to granulocytes (neutrophils, eosinophils, and basophils). Because determination of antigen presence on basophils and eosinophils is difficult, many antigens described as specific for neutrophils have not been tested for expression on nonneutrophilic granulocytes. For this reason, we will refer to these antigens as granulocyte-specific antigens, rather than by the more commonly used term, neutrophil-specific antigens.

The initial report of neutrophil-specific antigens was by Lalezari and co-workers in 1960,[10] who devised the convention for nomenclature of neutrophil antigens: N, for neutrophil-specific antigen, followed by a capital letter designating the locus of the gene controlling antigen production and a number designating a specific allele at that locus, eg, NA1, NA2. However, there have been a number of other antigens described that do not follow this convention.

Currently, there are at least 11 different loci described for genes producing granulocyte-specific antigens. Allelic genes producing antithetical antigens have been discovered at six of these loci. The granulocyte-specific antigens, their phenotype frequency, and their calculated gene frequencies are shown in Table 6–1.

NA NA1, which was defined by an antibody from a patient with neonatal neutropenia, was the first neutrophil-specific antigen to be described.[11] This antigen occurs on the granulocytes of approximately 46% of Caucasian blood donors. Lalezari and Radel[9] later showed that the antigen NA2 was the antithetical antigen to NA1. This relationship seems to be valid in the vast majority of families investigated. However, there are occasional exceptions noted to the inheritance of NA-locus antigens that hint that there may be a silent allele at the NA locus that produces neither NA1 nor NA2 antigens. This possibility was mentioned briefly by Lalezari[173] in connection with a family study he performed. We have recently observed a family with a mother whose granulocytes type as NA2/NA2 and a father whose granulocytes type as NA1/NA2. A son and a daughter type as NA2/NA2, but a second son types as NA1/NA1. None of the other blood groups tested in this family reveal any

Table 6-1.

Granulocyte-Specific Antigens

Locus	Antigens	Phenotype Frequency (%)	Genotype Frequency	Reference
NA	NA1	46	0.38	11,9,58
	NA2	88	0.63	173
NB	NB1	97	0.83	58,12
	NB2	32	0.17	61,174
NC	NC1	91	0.72	58,13
ND	ND1	98	0.88	60,179
NE	NE1	23	0.12	60,180
9	9a	58	0.35	60,364
HGA-3	HGA-3a	21	0.11	76
	HGA-3b	24	0.13	76
	HGA-3c	16	0.08	76
	HGA-3d	53	0.31	76
	HGA-3e	17	0.09	76
GA	A1,2,3,4,5	ND	ND	72
GB	B20,21,22,23,24	ND	ND	72
GC	C40,41,42,43	ND	ND	72
Gr	Gr1	ND	0.18	70
	Gr2	ND	0.35	70
Cold	Cold	100	ND	79,154
Group	Group 1	32	0.37	73
	Group 2	30	0.12	73
	Group 3	7	0.14	73
Group	Group 1	5	0.11	71
	Group 2	6	0.11	71
	Group 3	1	0.05	71
	Group 4	3	0.08	71
	Group 5	8	0.23	71

ABBREVIATION: ND = no data (pertains only to frequency data).
NOTE: Some variation in phenotype and genotype frequencies are noted among different populations studied.

other discrepancies and are entirely consistent with paternity. It appears that the mother's genotype is actually NA2/NA-, and that she passed the NA- gene to the second son, NA1/NA- and possibly to the other siblings as well (ie their genotype may be NA2/NA-). Attempts to determine true genotype with titration studies were not informative.

The NA antigens are truly neutrophil-specific as they have been shown to occur only on neutrophils (and not on eosinophils or basophils).[10,11]

NB Studies of fetomaternal incompatibility led Lalezari to describe the NB1 antigen in 1971.[12] It was shown to be neutrophil-specific and independent of the NA locus, and to have a gene frequency of 0.83. Until recently, NB1 was the only recognized antigen produced by alleles at this locus. In 1982, however, serum from a patient experiencing a febrile transfusion reaction was reported to contain an antibody defining NB2.[174] Anti-NB2 causing alloimmune neonatal neutropenia (ANN) was reported concurrently by Lalezari.[61] He not only showed the antigen to be neutrophil-specific and to have the expected gene frequency of 0.17, but also presented evidence that NB2 is identical to the 9a antigen (See 9 section).

Interest in this intriguing hypothesis linking the 9a antigen to the NB locus led us to examine our donor population for data to support it. In prospective GA testing of 281 donors in 1984, we found 14 donors (4.9%) that typed as negative for both NB1 and 9a. This data was inconsistent with simple allelism of NB1 and 9a. However, further recent testing of these and additional donors using GIF titrations and fluorescent flow cytometry have produced different results. Donors who initially appeared to lack both the NB1 and 9a antigens in GA testing actually expressed the NB1 antigen when tested by fluorescence methods. This data is consistent with 9a being identical to the NB2 antigen.

Further questions remain to be resolved, however. The increased sensitivity of fluorescence methods in detecting the NB1 antigen demonstrates a gene frequency of 0.85 in our donor population. When paired with that found for 9a in our study, 0.37, these antigens do not fit into as neat a biallelic system as was originally described by Lalezari. Also, we have found antibodies to 9a/NB2, including the original examples contributed to the NIH serum bank by van Rood (anti-9a) and Lalezari (anti-NB2), to react in only GA, not in GIF, as Lalezari reported.

NC NC1 was described in 1970,[13] defined by an antibody from a woman whose child was suffering from a mild case of alloimmune neonatal neutropenia. Her serum also contained a strong HLA antibody that reacted independently of the granulocyte antibody in the granulocyte agglutination assay. If the HLA activity is not removed by platelet absorption, misleading granulocyte testing results may occur. Although independent of the other neutrophil antigens, the NC1 antigen demonstrated a strong association with the NA2 antigen. This association was first noted by Lalezari in 1977[57] and later confirmed by Verheugt[175] and Schacter.[176] Additional studies by Schacter[177] indicated that the NC1 gene appeared to behave differently in blacks than in whites. She suggested that the genes controlling these two antigens segregated independently in blacks, but seemed to be identical in whites. However, such a discrepancy in gene activity among races is unprecedented.

We confirmed the strong NC1-NA2 relationship in a prospective study of normal, predominantly white blood donors using anti-NC1 (Vaz) absorbed with purified platelets to remove all the HLA antibodies.[178] We found three of 281 (1.1%) donors in which the NA2 and NC1 typings were not identical. All three of these donors had granulocytes that typed as NA2-positive, NC1-negative. These findings suggest to us that, although these two specificities are difficult to differentiate, they are not identical. The cells we found that typed as NA2-positive, NC1-negative failed to absorb anti-NC1, and therefore seem to truly lack the NC1 antigen. We currently believe that either the NA2 and NC1 antigens are produced by two tightly associated genes, or the NA2 antigen is a necessary precursor for the production of the NC1 antigen. If NA2 is a precursor of the NC1 antigen, one would expect that NA1/NA2 cells may have a decreased amount of the NC1 antigen when compared to NA2/NA2 cells. Titration studies performed in our lab tend to indicate that this is true (See chapter 7, Relationship of Zygosity and Strength of Antigen Expression).

ND Anti-ND1 was reported in 1978[179] by Verheugt et al. This specificity was defined in the sera of two patients who had autoimmune neutropenia. The analysis of families showed that this new specificity was not related to the NA, NB, NC, or 9a locus. The ND1 antigen was stated to be neutrophil-specific, although the results of cell line distribution studies were not reported. In tests on a small number of blood donors (n = 67), it was shown that the antigen was present on 98.5% of donors' neutrophils, corresponding to a gene frequency of 0.88, assuming a diallelic system.

NE Anti-NE1 was described in the serum of a child with chronic benign neutropenia.[180] The preliminary population analysis showed that there was no correlation between this antigen and the granulocyte-specific antigens NA1, NA2, NB1, NC1, and 9a. Its incidence in the Dutch population, again as determined by the tests on a small number (n = 48) of donors, was 23%, which corresponded to a gene frequency of 0.12.

Since this gene frequency hinted that NE1 might be the antigen produced by the allele of ND1 (gene frequency = 0.88), a series of families was examined to try to define this relationship. Two people were found whose granulocytes lacked both the ND1 and the NE1 antigen, indicating that they are not simply alleles.[181]

Using absorption tests, this antigen was shown to be only on granulocytes and not on lymphocytes, monocytes, platelets, or erythrocytes.

9 Reported by van Rood in 1965,[182] the 9a antigen was defined by an antibody in the serum of a multiparous donor. This antigen was shown to be present only on granulocytes and to have a gene frequency of 0.35.[364] Recently, Lalezari et al[61] presented evidence that 9a is actually the antithetical antigen to the NB1 antigen, and reported a gene frequency of 0.17.

HGA-3   Antibodies to the HGA-3 antigens described by Thompson et al[76] were detected and characterized using a double fluorochromatic granulocytotoxicity method. Population studies using these sera and this method have demonstrated five antigens that are produced by genes at this single locus. These antigens could be shown to be expressed on mature granulocytes, but not on platelets, lymphocytes, monocytes, and myeloid precursors. Since the gene frequencies of the HGA-3 antigen genes do not equal 1.00, there may still be some additional antigen produced at this locus. These antigens were shown to be independent of HLA, 5a-5b, NA, and NB. Only minute quantities of the sera used to define these antigens remain available; therefore, further investigation of this antigen system is prohibited due to reagent shortage.

GA, GB, and GC   Hasegawa and colleagues[72] described a series of studies using microgranulocytotoxicity that identified 14 specificities carried only on granulocytes. These antigens were produced at three loci that they called GA, GB, and GC. Although there was no association between these antigens and HLA or NA2 antigens, there was some ill-defined relationship detected with the NA1, NB1, and NC1 antigens. This relationship was not further characterized.

Gr   Caplan et al[70] described two antigens, defined by antibodies detected with a dye exclusion technique using cytochalasin-B–treated granulocytes. These two antigens were designated Gr1 and Gr2 and appeared to be the products of allelic genes. The antigens seemed to be present only on granulocytes. There was no apparent association with the HLA, NA, or NB antigens, but the authors said that these antigens may have been represented among those reported as being produced by the GA, GB, and GC loci described by Hasegawa.[72]

Maturation and Differentiation Antigens   Mahmoud et al[183] reported the production of monospecific antisera by injecting rabbits with purified suspensions of single-donor human granulocytes. They were successful in obtaining monospecific antisera against neutrophils, eosinophils, basophils, and myeloblasts. None of the antisera against mature cells reacted with myeloblasts, and conversely, the antisera against myeloblasts did not react with mature cells.

These experiments demonstrated that there are cell-specific antigens on each of the mature granulocyte lines that do not cross-react. They also pointed out that there are antigens present on myeloid precursors that are not present on mature cells, and conversely that there are antigens on mature granulocytes that arise after the myeloblast stage.

Antigens Defined by Cold-Reacting Antibodies Reported by both Lalezari[154] and Drew,[79] antibodies reactive primarily at lower temperatures were found to detect antigens present on all granulocytes (neutrophils, eosinophils, and basophils). These antigens were probably not related to the I or i antigens on red blood cells because they could be absorbed by either adult or cord red blood cells. However, like those against the I and i antigens, the antibodies occurred more commonly in patients following infection by Mycoplasma or infectious mononucleosis.

Groups 1, 2, and 3 Korinkova and co-workers[73] examined the sera of 904 multiply transfused or multiparous patients with a granulocytotoxicity test. They identified nine sera that did not contain lymphocytotoxins but defined three antigens that they designated group 1, group 2, and group 3. The antibodies appeared to detect antigens that only occurred on granulocytes, but absorptions were not reported with erythrocytes or platelets. The gene frequency of group 1 was calculated as 0.37, group 2 as 0.12, and group 3 as 0.14. The independence or relationship of these antigens to previously described granulocyte antigens was not reported.

Groups 1, 2, 3, 4, and 5 Using a modified granulocytotoxicity assay employing papainized granulocytes and a prolonged incubation period, Drew et al[71] identified five groups of reactions that defined five granulocyte antigens. The genes controlling the production of these antigens appeared to be allelic and had a combined gene frequency of 0.57 (group 1 = 0.11, group 2 = 0.11, group 3 = 0.05, group 4 = 0.08, and group 5 = 0.23). These antigens were not associated with HLA-A or HLA-B antigens or ABH antigens. By analyzing sibling pairs for the error rate for serologic reactions between HLA and these granulocyte antigens, it was shown that the rate was consistent with that expected when the two systems are located on different chromosomes and segregating independently.

Granulocyte-Monocyte Antigens

HGA-1 Thompson and colleagues [63,76,184] reported that the serum of patients immunized by bone marrow or kidney transplantation or multiple blood transfusions often contains antibodies that react with antigens common to monocytes and granulocytes. HGA-1 is an antigen that was shown to be present on granulocytes, myeloblasts, and monocytes, but was not demonstrated on platelets, lymphocytes, or red blood cells.[76] The gene controlling the production of this antigen was shown to segregate independently of HGA-3, NA, NB, and HLA. Absorption studies demonstrated that this serum contained a single antibody specificity because absorption with granulocytes removed all of the activity for monocytes and absorption with monocytes removed all of the activity for granulocytes.

AYD   Another antigen, defined by a serum designated AYD, was shown to be present on granulocytes, monocytes, and endothelial cells.[63] The gene controlling the production of the AYD antigen was shown to segregate independently from HGA-1, NA, NB, and HLA. Thompson has indicated the intriguing possibility that these antigens may prove to be another histocompatibility barrier, as they are associated with a higher rejection rate in patients who have had HLA-identical kidney transplants or bone marrow transplants from sibling donors.[63]

Systemic Antigens

Systemic antigens are defined as those antigens showing a wide tissue distribution and found on mature cells that are ontogenetically unrelated or only very distantly related. Systemic antigens can be divided into five main classes: (1) ABH antigens; (2) histocompatibility antigens; (3) antigens on erythrocytes and granulocytes; (4) antigens on monocytes, lymphocytes, and granulocytes; and (5) antigens on platelets, lymphocytes, and granulocytes.

ABH Antigens

Several groups of investigators reported the presence of ABH antigens on granulocytes.[57,156,185] These antigens were usually demonstrated on the surface of granulocytes by absorption studies. It may be significant that all of the studies detecting ABH antigens on granulocytes were performed prior to 1964 when the preparation of purified granulocyte suspensions was not well described. Therefore, the presence of white blood cells other than granulocytes in these preparations may have led to erroneous conclusions.

The study of ABH antigens on any type of circulating blood cells is further complicated by the fact that these antigens occur in a soluble form in plasma. Small amounts may be synthesized by plasma glycosyltransferases, which makes it difficult to determine whether the detected antigens are an integral part of the cell membrane or if they have been passively adsorbed onto the cell as it circulates in the plasma. It has been shown convincingly that platelets and red blood cells passively adsorb ABH antigens from the plasma.[186,187] This may be the reason that it is not possible to demonstrate the antigens on granulocytes by direct assays such as agglutination and cytotoxicity.

After repeated attempts in his laboratory to demonstrate ABH antigens on purified suspensions of granulocytes, Lalezari[157] reported failure to detect them using several methods: (1) opsonization when treated with high-titer anti-A and anti-B, (2) cytotoxicity measured by a variety of dye exclusion techniques, (3) the failure of granulocytes treated with anti-A and anti-B to support rosette formation with A and B erythrocytes. When they attempted to repeat their original absorption and elution experiments using highly purified granulocyte suspensions, they could not confirm their original results. This led them to conclude that the original suspensions of granulocytes were contaminated with a sufficient number of lymphocytes to cause the apparent absorption and subsequent elution of anti-A and anti-B.[157]

More recent attempts to show that granulocytes do carry the ABH antigens have been uniformly unsuccessful. McCullough and co-workers were unable to show any effect of anti-A and anti-B on the ability of indium 111–labeled granulocytes to survive in vivo or on their ability to localize at the site of infection.[188] This is very strong, suggestive evidence that there are not integral A and B antigens on granulocyte membranes because anti-A, anti-B, and anti-A,B are ordinarily very efficient at destroying transfused incompatible cells.

Karhi[189] recently showed that the A antigen (detected with the powerful anti-A lectin from *Vicia cracca*) could only be detected on bone marrow cells in the erythroid lineage. Neither erythroid cells earlier than the normoblast nor any other hematopoietic precursor cells showed the presence of A antigens.

In studies using human alloantibodies and mouse monoclonal antibodies against the A and B antigens, Dunstan et al[158,159] were not able to show any evidence that the A or B antigens are found on granulocytes with three separate techniques: (1) horseradish peroxidase cell labeling, (2) fluorescence flow cytometry, and (3) immunofluorescence microscopy. These assays appeared to be very sensitive and specific when used to test for other antigens on granulocytes.

Gaidulis et al[160] recently presented evidence using two assays that granulocytes do not express either the A or B antigens. They used an avidin-biotin complex immunoperoxidase cell staining method and an iodine 125–labeled staphylococcal protein binding assay. Although they used gluteraldehyde-treated granulocytes, they were able to show that these antigens were not denatured with a similar concentration of gluteraldehyde when used with red blood cells.

In summary, all recent investigations performed with pure preparations of granulocytes have overwhelmingly demonstrated the absence of ABH antigens on granulocytes. A variety of techniques have been used, including fluorescence flow cytometry, peroxidase labeling, immunofluorescence microscopy, iodine 125–labeled staphylococcal protein A, avidin-biotin complex immunoperoxidase staining, opsonization, cytotoxicity, rosette formation, anti-A lectin studies with bone marrow precursor cells, and in vivo indium 111 granulocyte kinetics and localization studies.

Human Leukocyte Antigens (HLA)

HLA-A and HLA-B (Class I) antigens can be demonstrated on the surface of granulocytes by absorption and elution studies,[64,190] agglutination,[191] and granulocyte immunofluorescence.[60] Attempts to demonstrate these antigens with granulocytotoxicity have been uniformly unsuccessful.[68,77,192] As previously described, HLA-A and HLA-B antigens and antibodies can be the cause of misleading and sometimes complex serologic results when working with assays to detect granulocyte-specific antigens or antibodies. Some of these complexities were described in a recent report by Clay et al.[164] Sera used for serologic or immunogenetic investigations with any of the commonly used granulocyte antibody assays must be carefully examined for the presence of HLA antibodies. When present, they must either be removed by absorption with purified suspensions of platelets or be used with granulocytes from donors known to lack the corresponding HLA antigens.

Class I HLA antigens appear to be present on granulocytes in significantly smaller quantities than those found on lymphocytes.[64] Lalezari et al[193] recently suggested that the HLA-A and HLA-B antigens found on platelets are passively adsorbed from the plasma. Although there is no direct evidence that the same is true of the Class I antigens on granulocytes, the recent demonstration that chloroquine removes HLA-A and HLA-B antigens from platelets and granulocytes while having no effect on cell-specific antigens may indicate that they are also passively adsorbed onto granulocytes.[136,137]

Although studies have shown that granulocytes can act as a stimulus for mitotic proliferation of lymphocytes in the mixed lymphocyte test,[194,195] those studies were performed prior to the introduction of highly purified cell suspensions. Therefore, conclusions regarding the presence of HLA-D (Class II) antigens cannot be drawn from these studies as activation may have been caused by contaminating lymphocytes in the preparations. Serologically defined Class II (Dr) antigens cannot be shown to occur on granulocytes by absorption.[63] Also, Dunstan[196] recently failed to show that granulocytes carry the Dr antigens by using mouse monoclonal antibodies directed against the Dr antigens in a fluorescence flow cytometer.

Granulocyte-Erythrocyte Antigens

The term "red blood cell antigens" in many cases is a significant misnomer. These antigens were in most cases found on red blood cells as a result of attempts to locate compatible red blood cells for transfusion. Because of the relatively early routine use of sensitive serologic techniques to detect red blood cell antibodies in compatibility testing and the common practice of red blood cell transfusions, there was a high possibility of producing and recognizing antibodies directed against antigens on red blood cells. Many of these antigens, therefore, were originally described as being carried on red blood cells and became known as red blood cell antigens by default. Often there was not a systematic attempt to determine whether they were also present on other cell lines. Interestingly, when there was more than one investigation to determine whether these antigens were on other cell lines, the evidence was often conflicting, depending upon the technique used. The results of newer techniques to demonstrate red blood cell antigens on granulocytes must be interpreted with caution until it can be determined how antibodies with different characteristics react in these assays. By analogy, anti-Jka would not be expected to cause the agglutination of saline-suspended red blood cells, while it will react quite well in the indirect antiglobulin test.

I/i The I and i antigens have been shown to be present on granulocytes by absorption and elution,[154] direct agglutination,[154] and granulocytotoxicity.[197,198] In addition, the i antigen was shown to be present on myeloid precursor cells by immunofluorescence.

Lewis The Lewis blood group antigens have been demonstrated on granulocytes by absorption and elution[199] but not by fluorescence flow cytometry.[159]

P In 1958 Archer[199] demonstrated the Tj^a antigen (P_1PPk) on granulocytes by absorption. Dunstan later confirmed this observation and also demonstrated that the P_1 and P antigens are on granulocytes using flow cytometry.[159]

MN Marsh[200] and Archer[199] were both able to demonstrate the U antigen on granulocytes by absorption and elution techniques. Neither group, however, was able to demonstrate any of the other MN system antigens. More recently, two additional investigators, Gaidulis[160] and Dunstan,[159] using flow cytometry, avidin-biotin complex staining, and iodine 125–labeled staphylococcal protein A, failed to demonstrate any of the MN system antigens, including U, on granulocytes.

Rh Although several groups of investigators have looked for Rh antigens on granulocytes by absorption and elution,[201] flow cytometry,[159] avidin-biotin complex cell staining, and iodine 125–labeled staphylococcal protein A,[160] only a single group[202] was able to find any evidence of Rh antigens.

Kell There are no reports of Kell antigens on granulocytes, although there have been several attempts to demonstrate them.[203–205] The Kx antigen, which is not produced by a gene at the Kell locus but is significantly associated with the Kell system because it produces a precursor of the Kell antigens on red blood cells, is found on all normal granulocytes.[205] In chronic granulomatous disease, the genetic lack of the Kx antigen from granulocytes is associated with a serious defect in granulocyte bactericidal function, which leads to susceptibility to life-threatening infections.[203,206]

Kidd   Marsh[207] was able to demonstrate Jk3 on granulocytes by absorption-elution; however, no other antigens in the Kidd system were demonstrable. More recently, Gaidulis[160] was not able to demonstrate any antigens in the Kidd system, including Jk3.

Duffy   None of the investigations of Duffy system antigens on granulocytes were able to produce any evidence that they are present.[159,201]

HTLA   The antigens usually recognized by HTLA (high-titer, low-avidity) antibodies (Chido, Rodgers, York, Cost-Stirling, Holley, Gregory, McCoy, JMH, Knops, or Sd[a]) are no longer regarded as occurring on granulocytes.[208]

Gerbich   Despite some recent evidence that Gerbich antigens are not found on granulocytes,[159,160] there is good evidence to the contrary. Gerbich antigens were shown by Marsh [209] to occur on granulocytes by absorption and elution techniques. Recently, we had the opportunity to repeat these absorption experiments while investigating a possible new phenotype in the Gerbich system. We were able to completely absorb anti-Ge1,2,3 and anti-Ge1,2 with normal Ge:1,2,3 granulocytes, but were not able to absorb these antibodies using granulocytes from Ge:−1,−2,−3 donors. In addition, when we tested 11 examples of sera containing Gerbich system antibodies in the granulocyte agglutination assay, we were able to show that nine of these sera reacted with granulocytes from Gerbich-positive donors. This is further evidence that granulocytes have Gerbich antigens on their surface.

Granulocyte-Monocyte-Lymphocyte Antigens

A new antigen was described in 1982[210] that had an unusual cell line distribution in that it was found on granulocytes (neutrophils, basophils, and eosinophils), monocytes, and lymphocytes, but was not demonstrable on erythrocytes or platelets. The antigen (called Mart) was defined by three examples of the antibody found in the sera of three nontransfused multiparous donors. The antigen was not associated with the granulocyte antigens NA1, NA2, NB1, NC1, ND1, NE1, or 9a, nor was it related to HLA or any of the common red blood cell antigens. The antigen was shown to have autosomal dominant inheritance. The sera reacted with 340 of 343 normal blood donors (99.1%), which corresponds to a gene frequency of 0.91. The significance of the antibody in mediating blood cell destruction is unknown, although none of the infants of these three women showed evidence of alloimmune neonatal neutropenia.

Granulocyte-Platelet-Lymphocyte Antigens

Van Leeuwen et al[211] reported a new diallelic system in 1964, which they designated group 5. This system consisted of two antigens, 5a and 5b. Antigen 5a had a gene frequency of 0.819 and 5b had a gene frequency of 0.181. These antigens have been reported to occur on granulocytes, lymphocytes, and platelets, and on kidney, placenta, and endothelial cells, but are not present on erythrocytes.[212,213] These antigens were independent of the HLA system, and recently they have been shown to be a product of genes located on the number 4 chromosome.[214]

Chapter 7

Characterization of Granulocyte Antigens

Very little is known about the hematopoietic myeloid expression of granulocyte-specific antigens. Furthermore, the physiochemical properties and biologic function of these antigens have not been established. Consequently, there is currently an interest in their isolation and chemical characterization.

Although the existence of alloimmune neonatal neutropenia implies expression of granulocyte antigens on infants' cells, a recent study by Madyastha et al[215] confirms this. They tested the granulocytes from cord blood taken from 33 black and 21 white newborns for NA1, NA2, NB1, NC1, and 9a. These were shown to be expressed in the infants to a degree that was not significantly different from that observed in adults, indicating that these granulocyte antigens are fully expressed in the newborn.

Antigen Expression

Using an immunofluorescence technique on bone marrow smears, Boxer et al[15] found the expression of the NA1 antigen to be restricted to myelocytes, metamyelocytes, bands, and mature neutrophils. Immunoelectron-microscopic studies by Verheugt and his associates have since suggested that the NA1, NB1, and ND1 antigens are present on myeloblasts, immature cells (promyelocytes, myelocytes, and metamyelocytes), and mature granulocytes.[59] No difference was seen in antigen density on mature granulocytes compared with granulocyte precursors. Further work needs to be done to expand the observations of these initial studies. However, successful engraftment of NA1-positive bone marrow in a patient with anti-NA1 suggested that granulocyte-specific antigens are not functionally present on the pluripotent stem cell.[216]

A unique feature associated with the NB1 antigen is its heterogeneous distribution on granulocytes.[59] NB1-positive granulocytes, when tested with anti-NB1, demonstrate three fluorescent patterns: strong, weak, and nonfluorescent (Figure 7–1). This has not been observed with the other granulocyte antigens. Verheugt's group found the heterogeneous expression also present on granulocyte precursors. They found no correlation of this interesting finding with homozygosity or heterozygosity for the x chromosome, or with morphological features of the granulocytes as determined by light microscopy.[59] We have found no correlation with homozygosity or heterozygosity of the NB1 antigen status, but we have observed genetic inheritance of the distribution density. Whether this distinct NB1 feature is identifying a granulocyte subpopulation remains to be seen. However, recent studies by Richards suggest that the NB1 antigen may be part of, or closely associated with, granulocyte membrane fMLP receptors,[217] which also demonstrate a heterogeneous profile.[218]

Figure 7–1.

Cytofluorometry histogram demonstrating the heterogeneous fluorescent labeling patterns of anti-NB1 with NB1-positive granulocytes. (A) No fluorescence, (B) weak fluorescence, (C) moderate to strong fluorescence.

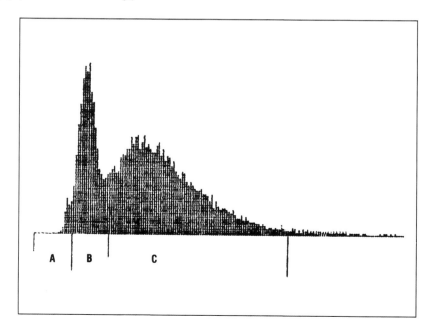

Monoclonal Antibodies

Numerous monoclonal antibodies recognizing myeloid-specific antigens have been reported.[106,219-228] These antigenic determinants are primarily myeloid differentiation and maturation markers. These antibodies have provided a mechanism for the understanding of granulopoietic differentiation with direct application to the study of myeloid leukemia. Some of them have also demonstrated the following abilities: (1) to inhibit granulocyte functions such as chemotaxis and degranulation[27] and superoxide production,[229] (2) to inhibit granulocyte Fc receptors for immunoglobulins and complement,[157,230] and (3) to specifically inhibit CFU-GM growth.[106] However, there have been no published reports of any myeloid monoclonal antibodies with specificity for the serologically defined granulocyte-specific antigens. We have had the opportunity to examine several monoclonal antibodies produced by Skubitz et al[224] and found no polymorphic serologic antibody specificities. Although the human promyelocytic leukemia cell line HL-60 is reactive with polyclonal rabbit antihuman granulocyte sera, the NA1, NA2, NB1, NC1, and ND1 antigens were not found to be present on this cell line.[220] Preliminary reports of monoclonal antibodies with granulocyte FcR activity and NA1 specificity have been presented by von dem Borne.[231] This finding has some very exciting possibilities but awaits further confirmation.

Immunochemistry

Although immunoprecipitation studies with myeloid monoclonal antibodies have identified polypeptides with molecular weights of 65K, 105K, and 150K daltons,[60] these have not been reported to be associated with serologically defined granulocyte-specific antigens. Thus far the only attempt to characterize granulocyte-specific antigens by immunoprecipitation has been carried out by Mulder.[232] One of two NB1 antibodies reacted with a 58,000 mol wt antigen present on NB1-positive granulocytes and absent from NB1-negative granulocytes. Anti-ND1 precipitated an antigen with a molecular weight of 55K daltons. Antibodies with NA1, NA2, and NC1 specificity failed to yield any bands. Although preliminary, this study reflects the current technology being used to explore the biochemical composition of granulocyte-specific antigens.

Relationship of Zygosity and Strength of Antigen Expression

Titration, a standard method of immunohematological investigation, provides a relatively easy method of quantitating antibodies and antigens. Because of the utility of this method and because we have found a need to evaluate the zygosity of test cells, we carried out a series of titrations with cells of known zygosity to determine whether granulocyte antigens exhibit dosage that could be measured by titrations with granulocyte antibodies.

We examined 22 cells of known zygosity with five granulocyte-specific antibodies. As seen in Table 7–1, antibodies against the NA1, NA2, and NB1 antigens showed a considerable area of overlap in the end point of titrations; however, there is a distinct correlation between the zygosity of the cells and the titer scores observed. This difference was not seen with the anti-NB2. While the allelic relationship of NB1 and NB2 has been reported,[61] confirming data has not followed. Interestingly, there was a difference in the strength of reactivity with anti-NC1 that was correlated with the NA locus zygosity. This is consistent with what would be expected if NA2 is a precursor of the NC1 antigen as suggested by Kline, et al.[178]

These results show that the titration strength of some examples of granulocyte-specific antibodies may be used to provide evidence as to the zygosity of granulocytes. Whether an antibody is suitable for these studies can be easily determined by testing it in titration with cells of known phenotype.

Disease Association

It is interesting to note that seven of the 14 (50%) cases of juvenile primary autoimmune neutropenia (AIN) reported in detail have been associated with NA1 autoantibodies.[21,233] Likewise, 16 of 32 (50%) sera from children with AIN and granulocyte-specific an-

Table 7–1. **Granulocyte Antigen Zygosity and Granulocyte Antibody Titrations**

Antibody		Homozygous Cells	Heterozygous Cells
Anti-NA1	Titer	4–32	2–8
	Mean score	39	29
Anti-NA2	Titer	4–32	2–4
	Mean score	39	22
Anti-NB1	Titer	64–>512	64–>512
	Mean score	42	33
Anti-NB2	Titer	64–128	16–128
	Mean score	47	47
Anti-NC1*	Titer	4–128	16–128
	Mean score	43	30

NOTE: All testing performed using the GA assay.
* Due to the observed correlation between NC1 and NA2, anti-NC1 was tested with homozygous and heterozygous NA2 cells.

tibodies referred to our laboratory for serologic evaluation were found to contain NA1 antibodies. The relatively high incidence of this antibody in this disease, in contrast with the gene frequency of NA1 in the general population (0.38), may some day provide a clue as to the function of this antigen and to the etiology of AIN.

A fascinating observation concerning the N series of granulocyte-specific antigens was made by Reijden and co-workers in 1979.[234] They measured the strength of the NA1, NA2, NB1, and ND1 with the indirect immunofluorescence assay in 23 patients with chronic granulocytic leukemia. Ten of the 23 patients studied showed a complete loss of all of these antigens, which correlated with an acceleration of their disease and progression to blast crisis.

Cell Line Distribution of Antigens

The presence or absence of granulocyte antigens on other cell lines may be closely related to their function and clinical significance. This important characteristic of granulocyte antigens is also one of the most difficult and time-consuming to investigate. There are now many different methods for determining which cell lines carry antigens, but one of the oldest and most sensitive is that of absorbing the serum with a preparation of purified cells. This method has the advantage of allowing the serum to be tested after absorption, thereby allowing one to determine with a fair degree of certainty whether or not the antibody in question is actually on the cells used for the absorption.

Because methods for absorbing sera are difficult and not readily available in the literature, the methods that we have found to be satisfactory in our laboratory are included in chapter 13.

Chapter 8

Genetics of Granulocyte Antigens

The study of granulocyte alloantigens presents an opportunity to describe and define new antigenic specificities. Alloantibodies to granulocytes in immunized transfusion recipients or multiparous females are a relatively common occurrence. However, there are only a few laboratories that are actively working with the granulocyte antibody assays in sufficient volume to develop the skills, antisera, and cell donors necessary to be able to fully characterize these antibodies. Cooperative efforts among other laboratories with more limited resources could provide valuable information on the genetics of new granulocyte antigens.

The following discussion will outline the procedures that we have found useful and necessary to characterize antibodies to granulocyte antigens and to explore the relationship between granulocyte alloantigens.

Population Studies

Testing unknown granulocyte alloantibodies with large numbers of random donors provides information critical to the characterization of new specificities.

Antigen Frequency

The frequency of occurrence of the antigen in a population is useful in several ways. First, it allows comparison of the frequency of an unknown antigen with that of previously described granulocyte antigens for possible identity. Second, it may provide clues as to possible association with known granulocyte antigens. Third, it may provide information as to association or identity with antigens described for other cell lines. Fourth, it allows calculation of the gene frequency, which permits more direct comparison with previously described antigens. Fifth, it will provide an accurate assessment of the difficulty of further investigations. Descriptions of antigens that are of extremely high or low incidence are exceedingly difficult to investigate.

Calculation of antigen frequency is straightforward:

$$\text{Antigen frequency} = \frac{\text{No. of samples expressing the antigen}}{\text{No. of samples tested for the antigen}}.$$

Two requirements are important to consider, however. First, any relatives of the antibody producer must be excluded from the count. Second, the minimum number of donors tested to make any meaningful estimate of the antigen frequency is 100, with 200 or more providing more reliable results. Random donors are the best sample. By testing the donors for other antigens with known frequencies and comparing the results, true randomness of the population may be assessed.

Gene Frequency

The gene frequency for newly described antigens may be calculated by a formula derived from the Hardy-Weinberg law, assuming a biallelic system and a population at equilibrium:

$$p = 1 - \sqrt{1 - Af},$$

where

  p = frequency of the gene that produces the antigen being studied
  Af = frequency of the antigen being studied (ie, all phenotypes)

Relationships with Known Antigens

When typing cells with an antibody to an unrecognized antigen, results must be systematically compared with typings for other known and unknown antigens.

We have found the most convenient method of arranging the data for the comparisons to be two-by-two contingency tables, as shown on the following page.

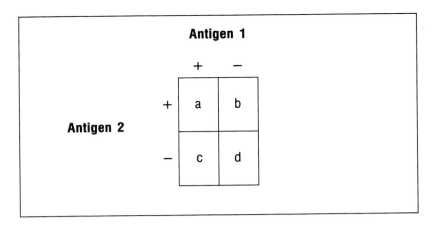

The relationship between two antigens can be easily determined and associations become obvious from examining the data. More importantly, it permits statistical evaluation of the relationship. We have found the following tests to be useful: (a) chi-square, (b) correlation coefficient, and (c) Fisher's exact method.

When looking for relationships with other antigens, it is important to be alert for identity, associations (statistically significant or suggestive evidence that antigens occur together more frequently or less frequently than expected), or an allelism.

Family Studies

Although a complete discussion of all of the intricacies of the interpretation of family studies and the elucidation of all of the genetics of granulocyte antigens is well beyond the scope of this book, a few of the principles and techniques that we have used in these studies will be presented here. Readers are referred to the texts of Cavalli-Sforza and Race and Sanger for excellent and comprehensive discussions of this subject.

Family studies involving granulocyte antigens present some specific problems which must be considered. In any family study, locating relatives in our modern, widespread society and making arrangements to have adequate samples drawn and shipped to the laboratory where testing is to be performed can be logistically challenging. However, this presents a major difficulty with granulocyte serology. As discussed previously, virtually all of the currently used granulocyte antibody assays require relatively fresh granulocytes. An additional complicating factor involves the advantages in testing all of the members of a family at the same time, whenever possible. This eliminates as many variables as possible in the testing and facilitates subsequent interpretation of the results.

Another difficulty is the sensitive issue of determining whether or not the individuals tested are really related as they believe they are. In order to answer this question, it is extremely important to test all of the individuals for well-described antigen systems, permitting exclusion of nonpaternity and nonmaternity. In our laboratory we routinely test for all of the common red blood cell antigens as well as for the generally recognized HLA-A and HLA-B antigens. These typings are critically important, both for assessing paternity and for subsequent comparisons for possible associations with the granulocyte antigens being tested.

Inheritance

Is the Antigen Inherited? One of the first observations to be made in family studies is whether or not the antigen being studied is inherited. This is usually easy to determine from the pattern of occurrence in the family. Antigens that have a very high incidence in the general population are more difficult to assess if the propositus is the only family member lacking the antigen. However, if the antigen has a very high incidence in the general population and is absent from parents and/or siblings of the propositus, its inherited character can be easily proven with common statistical methods (eg, chi-square). Proof of inheritance of antigens having a lower incidence in the population is also relatively easy. If the antigen occurs only in rare individuals in the population, but in a number of siblings and/or parents, then these antigens can likewise be shown statistically to be inherited.

Pattern of Inheritance In determining the pattern of inheritance of a characteristic, the first consideration should be whether the antigen is produced by a dominant or recessive allele. With rare exceptions, antigens found on various blood cells are controlled by codominant alleles. This implies that an antigen will be expressed on the cell for each allele carried. If an antigen is controlled by a dominant allele, at least one of the parents will also express the antigen on his or her cells. The proportion of siblings that will express the antigen varies depending on the zygosity of the parents with respect to the allele in question.

The second consideration in determining inheritance patterns is whether the allele controlling the production of the antigen in question is located on a somatic chromosome (autosomal linkage) or located on a sex chromosome (sex-linkage). Y-chromosome linkage is readily detectable (albeit rare) because the antigen will only be found in males. X-chromosome linkage gives a characteristic pattern of inheritance:

1. All of the daughters of a male expressing the antigen will express the antigen, regardless of the phenotype of the mother.

2. All of the sons of a male expressing the antigen with a mother lacking the antigen will also lack the antigen.

3. A mother heterozygous for the X-linked allele with a husband lacking the antigen will pass the allele to 50% of her sons and to 50% of her daughters.

Linkage

Determining linkage can be one of the most complex immuno-genetic projects. In the most comprehensive and exact manner, this requires performing a number of family studies and tabulating the number of recombinants and nonrecombinants between the gene for the antigen being studied and those of known antigens. After a sufficient number of families have been studied, a statistic called the "lod" (for *log of o*dds) score can be calculated or found in a table and the probability of linkage can be determined.

A much more inexact method is to observe recombination among siblings in a single family. Although this does not give the same level of confidence, recombinants seen in a single family can be taken as presumptive evidence that the two alleles being studied are not closely linked.

Evidence of Other Genetic Anomalies

Inhibitors and independent suppressors are rare but have been described for several antigen systems. They are relatively difficult to discern, but their hallmark is an antigen that was not apparent in either parent appearing in one or more of the offspring. When this is observed, nonpaternity must be first excluded on the basis of other antigen typings or another rare inherited trait. If this can be accomplished, then an inhibitor should be suspected as the cause.

Characterization of New Specificities

A number of antibodies detecting apparently undefined granulocyte antigens have been referred to our laboratory. From discussions with other investigators involved in granulocyte antibody testing, this is not an uncommon finding. The antigens defined by these unknown antibodies may be associated with functional properties of granulocytes or associated with clinically significant immune neutropenias. For these reasons and because these antigens may also play a useful role in some of the other traditional uses for immunohematology (eg, paternity studies, population genetic studies, disease associations, and transplantation), the effort required to thoroughly investigate them is merited. Unfortunately, the adequate characterization of antigens is a time-consuming process, and therefore it is often incomplete or done on an insufficient number of samples to be totally accurate.

The purpose of this section is to outline the minimum criteria necessary to accurately characterize a new granulocyte antigen.

I. SELECTION OF SERA FOR INVESTIGATION

Purpose: To ascertain if a serum sample contains an antibody defining a previously undescribed antigen.

Method:

1. Test the serum sample against a minimum of 20 granulocyte samples that have been typed for all of the common granulocyte-specific antigens (NA1, NA2, NB1, NB2, NC1, ND1, 9a, and Mart).

2. Titrate the antibody whenever possible; sera to be investigated should have a titer of at least 16.

3. Test for lymphocytotoxic antibodies. Nonreactivity simplifies further characterization of the granulocyte antibody.

4. Assess the volume of serum available and/or the potential for obtaining additional serum. Extremely small quantities may limit the accuracy of the original investigation and the possibility for future collaboration with other laboratories.

Analysis:

1. Set up two-by-two contingency tables plotting the reactivity with the new serum against each of the common granulocyte-specific antigens.

2. Calculate a chi-square, Fisher's exact, and correlation coefficient statistic for each of the contingency tables.

3. If there is no suggestive association ($p < .100$) between the reactions of the serum being investigated and the granulocyte antigens expressed on the panel, then the serum should be investigated.

II. IDENTIFICATION OF OTHER BLOOD GROUP ANTIBODIES

Purpose: To identify alloantibodies directed against blood cells other than granulocytes. Presence of such antibodies must be considered for potential interference in some granulocyte assays and absorbed when necessary. They may also provide information regarding the specificity of the granulocyte antibody.

Red Blood Cell Antibodies

Method: Perform a red blood cell antibody screening using two cells selected for their content of all of the common red blood cell antigens. Tests should be incubated at both 20°C and 37°C, taking 37°C tests through the antiglobulin phase.

Analysis: If red blood cell antibodies are present, the granulocyte panel donors should be typed for all of the common red blood cell antigens. The pattern of the reactive cells should be carefully examined to determine if the granulocyte antibody has a specificity identical or related to the corresponding red blood cell antibody.

Lymphocytotoxic (HLA) Antibodies

Methods:

1. Test for lymphocytotoxins against HLA-A, HLA-B, and HLA-C locus antigens using a 20-cell panel of selected lymphocytes in the standard NIH microlymphocytotoxicity assay.

2. Test for lymphocytotoxins against Dr locus antigens using a panel of ten selected B-lymphocytes in the standard lymphocytotoxicity method.

Analysis: If HLA antibodies are present, then the serum should be absorbed with pooled platelets until it is nonreactive with the lymphocyte panel. Absorbed serum should then be used for all further granulocyte antibody studies.

Platelet-Specific Antibodies

Method: Test for platelet-specific antibodies using a panel of five selected platelet samples in the platelet immunofluorescence assay.

Analysis: If platelet-specific antibodies are present, the granulocyte panel donors should be typed for the common platelet-specific antigens. The pattern of reactivity should be carefully examined to determine whether the granulocyte reactivity is identical or related to the platelet-specific antibody.

III. PHENOTYPIC ASSOCIATION

Purpose: To evaluate possible relationships between the antigen being investigated and any of the other commonly recognized blood cell antigens.

Method: Test the serum containing the unknown antibody with a minimum of 50 panel cells that have been typed for the following antigens:

1. Granulocyte-specific antigens: NA1, NA2, NB1, NB2, NC1, ND1, 9a, and Mart.

2. HLA antigens: HLA-A, HLA-B, HLA-C, and Dr antigens.

3. Red blood cell antigens: A, B, D, C, c, E, e, M, N, S, s, Le^a, Le^b, Fy^a, Fy^b, Jk^a, Jk^b, K, and k.

Analysis:

1. Arrange the results on a series of two-by-two contingency tables.

2. Test the data for association using the chi-square and correlation coefficient.

3. Any p value of less than .10 obtained with the chi-square, or any correlation coefficient greater than .65 or less than

−.65 should be considered sufficient evidence to test an additional 25 fully phenotyped donors with reanalysis as listed in Analysis steps 1 and 2 above.

4. This analysis is designed to detect the following:

   a. identity

   b. allelism/antitheticalism

   c. associations

   d. independence

IV. FREQUENCY OF OCCURRENCE

Purpose: To establish the antigen frequency and the gene frequency in a random population.

Methods:

1. Make a preliminary estimate of the occurrence of the antigen from the initial studies performed to determine the number of tests with random donors needed to obtain the 95% confidence level. Calculate the number of donors necessary to test from Figure 8–1. The D in the figure refers to the distance. Distance is a range in percent that corresponds to the 95% confidence level. For example, D = 10 means that the sample size is sufficient that the result will be plus or minus 10% with confidence of 95%.

2. Test the required number of donors using the appropriate granulocyte antibody assay.

Analysis:

1. Calculate the antigen frequency (Af) by dividing the number of reactive samples by the total number of donors tested.

2. Calculate the gene frequency, assuming that the antigen is produced by one allele of a biallelic system, using the formula $p = 1 - \sqrt{1 - Af}$.

3. Compare the gene frequency and antigen frequency with those of the common granulocyte-specific antigens to determine whether there is a close correspondence. Consider the possibility that the antibody is recognizing an allele to one of the previously described granulocyte-specific antigens by comparing the value $1.0 - p$ for correspondence to any of the gene frequencies.

V. INHERITANCE

Purpose: To determine if and how the antigen is inherited.

Figure 8-1.

Plots for the equation for determining the number of donors that need to be tested to establish the antigen frequency in a population with 90% confidence at three different distances. Distance is a range in percent that corresponds to the 95% confidence level.

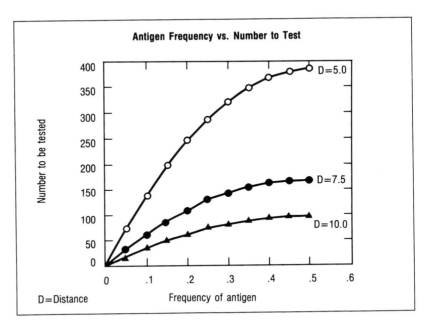

Method:

1. If possible, carefully select for investigation a family that represents three generations. At least one member of the family must lack the antigen being investigated.

2. Type the family for all of the common red blood cell, HLA-A, HLA-B, HLA-C, Dr, and granulocyte-specific antigens.

3. Chart the results on a pedigree diagraming the family relationships.

Analysis: Review the family study data for evidence to answer the following questions regarding the gene controlling the production of the antigen under investigation:

1. Does it act as a dominant or recessive allele?

2. Is it carried on a sex chromosome or on an autosome?

3. Is there evidence of its independence from the genes of other blood cell antigens (eg, recombination)?

4. Is there evidence of its linkage with those of other blood cell antigens?

VI. CELL TYPINGS OF THE ANTIBODY PRODUCER

Purpose: To exclude or focus on possible antibody specificities using the red blood cell, granulocyte-specific, and HLA types of the antibody producer.

Method: Type the cells of the antibody producer for all of the granulocyte-specific, red blood cell, and HLA antigens using standard techniques.

Analysis:

1. If the antibody being investigated is an alloantibody, its specificity cannot be identical to any of the antigens present on the patient's cells. (The possibility of mosaicism must be considered, but it is generally obvious.)

2. The antibody being investigated will be excluded from belonging to any known biallelic system if the patient is heterozygous for any of these systems.

3. If the patient's cells lack either a high-incidence antigen or lack both antigens of a biallelic system, special attention should be directed to determining if the antibody is related to these systems.

VII. CELL LINE DISTRIBUTION

Purpose: To identify the blood cell lines expressing the investigated antigen.

Method:

1. Identify cell lines that carry the antigen by performing absorption studies with the following purified cell suspensions from donors whose granulocytes react with the serum being investigated.

  a. erythrocytes

  b. platelets

  c. lymphocytes

  d. monocytes

2. Retest the unabsorbed and absorbed serum in parallel with a selected granulocyte sample by titrating it in the appropriate granulocyte antibody assay.

Analysis: If the serum no longer reacts with the granulocytes after absorption, then the antigen is considered to be carried on the absorbing cell line. If the serum is still reactive at the same titer after the absorption, then the antigen is not present on that cell line. Significant reduction in titer (fourfold or greater) suggests the presence of the antigen on the cell line and merits further studies.

VIII. CLINICAL SIGNIFICANCE

Purpose: To evaluate the antibody being investigated for any capability of causing functional impairment or in vivo destruction of granulocytes.

Method:

1. The patient should be personally interviewed if possible.

2. All of the available written medical records should be carefully reviewed.

Analysis: The patient's medical history should be investigated thoroughly to determine whether there is evidence of alloimmune or autoimmune neutropenias, transfusion reactions, or significant infections.

Exclusion of Antigens Defined by Rare Antisera

Numerous antigens described over the years are defined by sera that have not been widely distributed among laboratories involved in granulocyte antibody testing, or are no longer available for use in investigations. Whether due to antibody producers who are inaccessible for further donations or to changes in primary interests of investigators, laboratories interested in describing new granulocyte antigens are placed in the difficult position of trying to establish an apparently new specificity without being able to test for previously described antigens. In addition, there is the difficult problem of antigens defined by assays unique to a single laboratory that cannot be (or are not) performed in any other laboratory.

We believe that these problems are a major impediment to the description of a number of antigens. Consequently, we feel that if sera describing these antigens are not available for distribution or if the identity of the new antigen cannot be included from the previously described antigens by the reporting investigators, then it is not necessary to exclude the previously described antigens in the description.

Of course, if it is obvious that the newly investigated antigen is the same or related to the previously described antigens (through relationships to other well-recognized antigens, antigen frequency, or other testable parameters), then this should be acknowledged.

Chapter 9

Clinical Significance of Granulocyte Antigens and Antibodies

Neutropenia may be caused by a number of factors, both nonimmune and immune, resulting in decreased production or increased destruction of neutrophils (Table 9–1). However, in most patients neutropenia is attributable to nonimmune mechanisms. Failure of production due to iatrogenic factors such as chemotherapy, irradiation therapy, or as an idiosyncratic reaction to drugs are probably the most common causes of neutropenia.

Immunologic processes may also cause neutropenia due to decreased production or accelerated destruction. Alterations in T-cell and B-cell number or function, or antibodies against myeloid precursor cells, are examples of immunologic decreases in neutrophil production. These are complex processes which are not well understood. This discussion will focus on accelerated destruction of more mature neutrophils. This occurs predominantly by antibody-mediated mechanisms, but there will be some discussion of cell-mediated destruction of mature granulocytes. Much of the information about the clinical significance of granulocyte-specific antibodies is derived from studies of neutropenic patients. The clinical effects of these antibodies can be considered by separating problems caused by alloantibodies from those due to autoantibodies.

Clinical Problems Due to Alloantibodies

Alloimmune Neonatal Neutropenia (ANN)

The best-understood of situations involving granulocyte-specific alloantibodies, ANN is the neutrophil analogue of red blood cell he-

Table 9-1.   General Classification of Causes of Neutropenia

Decreased Neutrophil Production	Abnormal release from marrow
	Bone marrow suppression (toxicity)
	Idiopathic
	Idiosyncratic drug reaction
	Infection/sepsis
	Nutritional deficiencies
	Progenitor cell disorders
	Acquired
	Inherited
	Replacement of normal marrow
	Stem cell disorders
	Inherited
	Acquired
	T- and B-cell disorders
	Toxic injury
Increased Neutrophil Destruction	Alloimmune neonatal neutropenia
	Autoimmune neutropenia
	Primary
	Secondary
	Complement activation
	Disease
	Drugs
	Immune complexes
	Infection
Maldistribution of Neutrophils	Pseudoneutropenia

Source: Adapted with permission of McGraw-Hill from Lichtman MA: Classification of neutrophil disorders, in William WJ (ed): *Hematology*, 3rd ed. New York: McGraw-Hill, 1983, pp 770–772.

molytic disease of the newborn. Fetal cells cross the placenta during pregnancy and immunize the mother. Since granulocytes are motile cells, this transplacental passage may be active and not due to a placental defect.[235] IgG antibodies formed by the mother then cross the placenta to cause neutropenia in the infant. Although the incidence of neutrophil immunization is estimated as only 0.1% in multiparous women,[164] as many as two in 1,000 live births, and 1.5% of all admissions to a neonatal special care unit, have been reportedly associated with ANN.[236] Neonates are protected from infection in utero but may develop infections during the first few days of life. Often the infections are mild and include skin infections, omphalitis, otitis, fever, and respiratory or urinary tract infections.[9] However, serious infections can occur, causing a mortality from ANN of approximately 5%.[235] ANN is usually treated successfully with antibiotics, and corticosteroids are not indicated. Exchange transfusion could remove the offending antibody in some cases. The patients recover spontaneously in 2 weeks to 6 months as the maternal IgG antibody is catabolized and the neutrophil count returns to normal as demonstrated in one patient we followed (Figure 9–1). Antibodies in ANN are usually detected by granulocyte agglutination (GA), although some have been identified by granulocyte immunofluorescence (GIF).[9,17,57,59,235] It is not known whether antibodies detected only by GIF are weak examples that, if stronger, would be detected by GA, and whether these differences relate to the clinical effect of the antibodies. The antibodies most commonly involved are NA1 and NB1.[235]

Transfusion Reactions

Several pioneering studies established that febrile nonhemolytic transfusion reactions are caused by leukocyte antibody-antigen reactions.[217,302] This was based on the following evidence: (1) Use

---

Figure 9–1.

Total leukocyte and neutrophil levels relative to anti-NA1 levels in a patient with alloimmune neonatal neutropenia.

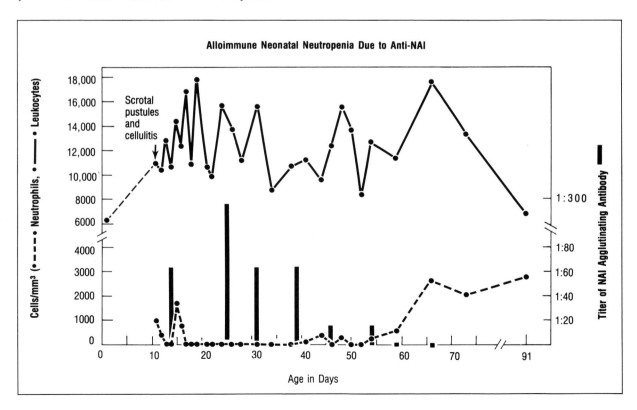

of red blood cells from which white blood cells had been removed eliminated the reactions, (2) infusion of as little as 50 mL of plasma containing white blood cell antibodies caused the febrile transfusion reaction, and (3) a statistical association between white blood cell antibodies and febrile transfusion reactions. Most of the reactions were thought to be due to antibodies in the recipient reacting with transfused incompatible leukocytes.[7,237]

Febrile Initial studies of leukocyte antibodies in febrile transfusion reactions were done using leukoagglutination. Although there was a general association between the presence of leukoagglutinins and occurrence of transfusion reactions, as many as one third of patients with reactions did not have leukoagglutinins.[7] This suggests either that some febrile transfusion reactions have other causes, or that the antibody detection techniques are not ideal. Many leukocyte antibody methods have been developed since those early studies; however, there are few studies comparing the value of different methods in predicting a febrile transfusion reaction. Thus, even today the best in vitro serologic method to predict a febrile transfusion reaction is not known. It is still not clear whether this is due to inadequate serologic tests or whether some reactions have other causes.

The clinical signs and symptoms of a febrile transfusion reaction, which were characterized almost 30 years ago by Brittingham and Chaplin,[238] include immediate, latent, and delayed phases (Table 9–2). These transfusion reactions occur frequently following red blood cell transfusions, but often may not be reported to the blood bank. Because hemolysis is not involved, unfortunately blood bankers may not consider such reactions very important even when

Table 9–2.   **Clinical Characteristics of Leukocyte-Mediated Transfusion Reactions**

Immediate Phase	Latent Phase	Delayed Phase
Onset ∼5 min	15–16 min	Onset ∼1 h
Flush	No symptoms	Headache
Palpitation		Chills
Tachycardia		Increased diastolic blood pressure
Cough		Fever
Choking		Rigors
Neutropenia		Irritability
		Confusion
		Apathy
		Leukocytosis

SOURCE: Brittingham TE, Chaplin H: Febrile transfusion reactions caused sensitivity to donor leukocytes and platelets. *JAMA* 165:819–825, 1957.

they are reported. When a reaction occurs, there is considerable discomfort and concern on the part of the patient; nursing and physician staff time is required to attend the patient and manage the reaction; the desired red blood cell transfusion is interrupted and delayed; and work is created for the blood bank to carry out the investigation of possible hemolysis. Thus, cost-effective approaches to preventing these reactions would be valuable contributions to improved transfusion therapy.

Pulmonary   The most severe form of a leukocyte transfusion reaction is the acute, sometimes fatal, pulmonary reaction, noncardiac pulmonary edema. These reactions are characterized by dyspnea, hypoxia, and infiltrates on chest roentgenogram. Since only 25 reported cases were found by Popovsky et al[239] they seem to be relatively rare. However, several descriptions in the older literature of leukocyte reactions sound similar to these cases.[240] It has been suggested that many pulmonary reactions attributed to hypervolemic pulmonary edema, infusion of cellular debris (microaggregates), or allergy (IgA deficiency) are in fact due to leukocytes. This is supported by the report of five cases from the Mayo Clinic where careful follow-up showed that the incidence of these reactions was 0.02% per unit or 0.16% per patient.[239]

Most pulmonary reactions have been associated with leukoagglutinating antibodies,[23,67,239-242] although some have involved lymphocytotoxins.[239,241] Even more striking, however, is that most of these cases of severe pulmonary reactions involve the passive transfusion of the offending antibody in donor plasma. This is markedly different from the usual situation with febrile nonhemolytic reactions, in which the recipient's antibody reacts with donor leukocytes. This situation was first described by Brittingham in 1957,[238] who reported that transfusion of 50 mL of whole blood to a normal subject caused vomiting, diarrhea, chills, fever, dyspnea, tachypnea, hypotension, and cyanosis. The subject developed marked pulmonary infiltrates on roentgenogram. Transfusions of plasma containing leukocyte antibodies from patients with autoimmune granulocytopenia,[243] drug-related granulocytopenia,[6] Felty's syndrome,[244] and granulocytopenia following mycoplasmal pneumonia[245] have caused neutropenia and severe clinical symptoms in recipients including dyspnea and cyanosis, although chest roentgenograms were not done on most patients. Thus, there is some indication that the more frequent and generally more mild febrile transfusion reactions may be associated with antibody in the recipient, while the severe pulmonary reactions may be associated with transfusion of donor antibody.

The pathophysiologic method by which transfusion of a relatively small amount of antibody causes such a severe clinical problem is not well understood. It seems likely that these antibodies initiate some type of amplification mechanism, probably complement activation. Complement activation, with resulting production of C5a and its attachment to the granulocyte, alters the cell membrane causing granulocytes to adhere nonspecifically to many different surfaces.[246] These cells are sequestered primarily in the pulmonary vascular bed,[247-249] where they become activated, releasing proteolytic enzymes and toxic oxygen metabolites.[247] It has been postulated that this sequence, with the combination of complement activation, neutrophil activation with enzyme release, and production of toxic oxygen metabolites, leads to acute lung injury.[250] Pulmonary sequestration of granulocytes could cause further endothelial damage and also lead to microvascular occlusion. Several clinical situations provide further support for the role of complement activation in this process. Complement activation, generation of C5a, and pulmonary sequestration of granulocytes occur when blood comes in contact with hemodialysis membranes or nylon fibers (filtration leukapheresis). This process is associated with transient neutropenia and pulmonary dysfunction.[251] We have described a patient who had a severe pulmonary reaction following transfusion of approximately 100 mL of the granulocyte antibody, anti-NA2.[23] Incubation of this antibody with material from the aortic graft that the patient was receiving at the time of transfusion caused complement activation in vitro.

Optimum serologic methods to detect and prevent severe pulmonary reactions have not been defined, but that the problem is more likely to be due to donor rather than recipient antibody. Some authors[241] have even suggested that blood from multiparous or multitransfused donors should be used only as packed red blood cells.

Granulocyte Transfusions

The development of granulocyte transfusions spurred interest in establishing in vitro tests to detect immune destruction of granulocytes, allowing donor-recipient matches to provide safe and effective transfusions. Early reports suggested that HLA matching provided satisfactory granulocyte increments posttransfusion.[252,253] However, almost all patients studied had both lymphocytotoxic and leukoagglutinating antibodies, so the relative role of HLA and granulocyte-specific antigens could not be distinguished. Also, the increases in granulocyte count being measured were usually less than 500 per μL, and such changes in infected neutropenic patients may not be accurate. In separate studies, others did not observe differences in the clinical improvement of patients regardless of the presence or absence of leukocyte incompatibility. Subsequent experience did not substantiate the initial optimism that leukoagglutinin or lymphocytotoxic antibody testing provided satisfactory in vitro matching for granulocyte transfusion.[254] One major problem has been the lack of a satisfactory method to study the fate of granulocytes in vivo and to determine whether an individual granulocyte transfusion is successful. We have tried to overcome this problem by developing a technique for labeling granulocytes with indium 111 (see chapter 10). Also, present granulocyte serologic techniques are not practical for crossmatching. They are complex, and time-consuming, and most require fresh viable granulocytes.[255] Since granulocyte concentrates are not a stock component, no fresh cells are routinely available for crossmatching, and carrying out a crossmatch would necessitate calling in donors. Even after this extra effort, the serologic tests are cumbersome, and the process of selecting donors and processing the granulocyte concentrate could take 2 days. As a result, there is no generally accepted approach to donor-recipient matching or leukocyte compatibility testing for granulocyte transfusions. This has become a smaller problem in the past few years as the use of granulocyte transfusions has declined. However, it also seems likely that lack of suitable techniques to provide a compatible granulocyte transfusion contributes to the lack of effectiveness of granulocyte transfusion.

Transplantation

Organ Transplantation Thompson[63] reported a series of 31 patients receiving HLA-identical, MLC-nonreactive kidney transplants. Serum samples were examined pretransplant, 1 month posttransplantation, and either at posttransplant nephrectomy or 3 to 6 months after transplantation. The sera were examined for cytotoxins against T-cells, B-cells, monocytes, and granulocytes. There was a significant increase in the number of patients producing granulocyte-monocyte cytotoxins who rejected the graft or died when compared to the patients with successful grafts.

There was also a significant association between the production of these antibodies and prior blood transfusions. Granulocyte-monocyte antibodies appeared in eight of the 16 patients who had received no blood transfusion prior to surgery. In these patients the antibodies were associated with either rejection of the transplant or a severe rejection episode. Of the 15 patients transfused prior to surgery, only four produced granulocyte-monocyte antibodies. These were not associated with a severe rejection episode, and only one of the patients rejected the kidney.

Thompson[63] suggested that these data and those of other groups[256-258] indicate that non-HLA granulocyte and monocyte antigens may serve as significant histocompatibility barriers in organ transplantation.

Bone Marrow Transplantation Granulocyte alloantibodies might also be important in bone marrow transplantation if granulocyte-specific antigens are on hematopoietic precursor cells, as the presence of circulating antibody in the recipient could interfere with granulocyte engraftment. It appears, however, that this is not so. NA1-positive bone marrow was successfully engrafted in a patient with anti-NA1.[216] However, as expected, mature granulocytes did not appear in the circulation until the remaining granulocyte antibody had been catabolized.

Clinical Problems Due to Autoantibodies

Primary Autoimmune Neutropenia (AIN)

Clinical Features   There were many reports during the 1950s describing studies of granulocytopenic patients. Although it is difficult to determine whether those patients should be included in this summary, the reports are quite valuable. One particular patient reported in detail seems to fit the present description of autoimmune granulocytopenia.[243] It is of particular interest that transfusion of the patient's plasma into a normal subject caused chills, fever, and a decrease in leukocytes and granulocytes. Neutropenia in these patients was thought to have an immunologic basis, but the cause was not established. Leukocyte antibodies were sometimes present but not always sought. Then, in 1975 Lalezari[173] and Boxer et al[19] showed that antigranulocyte antibodies were associated with neutropenia and reacted with the patient's own cells, and that the neutrophil level returned to normal when the antibodies disappeared. We have since documented similar cases,[29] and it is now established that primary AIN is caused by autoantibodies against granulocyte-specific antigens.

Patients with primary AIN have neutropenia as their only hematologic abnormality, without associated diseases or factors that might be the cause of the neutropenia.[259,260] Thirty-two patients who appeared to have autoimmune neutropenia without another underlying disease were reported in some detail (Table 9–3). Eighteen of these were children; 13 were females and all were 2 years old or less. These patients had infections of mild to moderate severity, most commonly otitis or infections involving the skin (boils, cellulitis), oropharynx, and upper respiratory tract. A few children developed pneumonia while others had very mild infections that did not require treatment. It has been postulated that a compensatory monocytosis may account for the mild to moderate nature of the infections, but monocytes were not increased in most of these cases (Table 9–4). The 14 adults ranged from 20 to 72 years in age, and there was a preponderance of females. Infections in the adults, as in the children, ranged from none to rather severe, but tended to be mild. The areas involved were usually the skin and oropharynx. It has been suggested that, on the basis of laboratory data, AIN can be classified as benign or complicated.[261] Peripheral blood neutrophil counts greater than 500 per microliter, response to a steroid challenge test, and normal or slightly decreased bone marrow myeloid elements predict a benign clinical course. Peripheral blood neutrophil counts less than 500 per microliter, lack of response to a steroid challenge test, and decreased bone marrow myeloid elements predict a complicated clinical course.

Table 9–3.   **Clinical Aspects of Patients with Primary Autoimmune Neutropenia**

Reference	Age	Sex	Nature of Infection	Treatment	Response
Lalezari et al[173]	2 yr	F	Otitis, respiratory, rash	Steroids	Yes
Boxer et al[19]	20 yr	M	Stomatitis, cellulitis	Steroids	Yes
	72 yr	F	Pharyngitis, meningitis	Splenectomy	Temporary
	3 mo	F	Boils, otitis, pharyngitis	Steroids	Yes
	45 yr	F	None	Splenectomy	Yes
	50 yr	F	None	Steroids	Yes
Valbonesi et al[365]	8 mo	F	Otitis, pneumonia, pyoderma	Steroids	Yes
Verheugt et al[82]	69 yr	M	Pneumonia	None	No
	2 yr	F	Pneumonia, otitis	Steroids	Yes
Lightsey et al[363]	45 yr	F	None	Steroids	Yes
Cline et al[117]	28 yr	F	Pyelonephritis	Steroids, cyclophosphamide, splenectomy	Yes
McCullough et al[29]	7 mo	F	Mild	None	Yes
	18 mo	M	Mild	None	Yes
Claas et al[180]	3–6 mo	NR	Respiratory	NR	NR
	3–6 mo	NR	Otitis	NR	NR
	3–6 mo	NR	Mastoiditis	NR	NR
Thompson et al[233]	7 mo	F	Cough, fever, otitis, diarrhea	Steroids	Yes
Nepo et al[366]	3 mo	F	Furuncles, otitis, fever	Steroids	Yes
Madyastha et al[367]	10 mo	F	None	None	NR
Kay et al[368]	5 mo	F	Respiratory	NR	NR
Blashke et al[77]	28 yr	M	Abscess, fever, night sweat, arthralgia, oral ulcers	Steroids, splenectomy	Yes—very little; later developed Hodgkin's disease
Smith et al[65]	56 yr	F	None	None	Yes
Bom van Noorloos et al[110]	58 yr	M	Ulcers of oropharynx and skin, diverticulitis	None	Died
Caligaris-Cappio et al[166]	67 yr	F	Skin	Splenectomy	Stable
	69 yr	M	Skin and urinary tract	Steroids, plasma exchange	Yes
	35 yr	F	None	None	Yes
Carmel[369]	34 yr	F	Fever, pharyngitis, adenopathy	Steroids	Yes
Sabbe et al[370]	5 mo	M	Mastoiditis	None	NR
	7 mo	F	Mastoiditis	None	NR
	8 mo	M	None	None	NR
	8 mo	M	Bronchitis	None	NR
	8 mo	M	Bronchitis	None	NR
Freed[336]	64 yr	F	Skin abscess, oral ulcers	Cyclophosphamide	Yes

ABBREVIATION: NR = not reported.

Laboratory Observations in Primary AIN The total leukocyte count in these patients ranged from normal to 1,000 per microliter (Table 9–4). Most patients had neutrophil levels less than 1,000 per microliter, and many were very low. There was usually a normal number of lymphocytes, although the percentage was increased due to the lack of neutrophils. Although a monocytosis has been reported in patients with primary AIN, monocytes were not increased in most of these patients. The bone marrow cellularity ranged from normal to hypercellular. Most patients had a decrease in some forms of myeloid elements, and erythroid and megakaryocytic elements were normal. There was usually an absence of mature granulocytes and band forms. While bone marrows in many patients with primary AIN are interpreted as showing a "maturation arrest," the absence of mature myeloid forms is caused by immunologic destruction rather than interference with maturation. Harmon et al[262] have shown that the degree of neutropenia increases as sera react with earlier myeloid forms. They postulated that antibodies that react only with more mature cells cause neutropenia only if the marrow response is inadequate. Antibodies that also react with earlier forms reduce the marrow response and cause more severe neutropenia.

Leukocyte Serology Antibodies reactive against most of the known granulocyte-specific antigens have been implicated in primary AIN, and react in a variety of leukocyte antibody assays (Table 9–4). It is not possible to extrapolate from this data which assay, if any, are more effective since most patients were tested by only one or two assays. In two patients we found that granulocyte-agglutinating, but not granulocytotoxic, activity was related to neutropenia.[29]

Therapy Initial treatment of these patients involves management of any infection present with antibiotics and other appropriate efforts. Therapy directed toward improving the neutrophil count has involved the use of corticosteroids, splenectomy, and, more recently, intravenous immune globulin. Six of the children reported with primary AIN were treated with steroids and all responded (Table 9–3); however, long-term follow-up is not reported for most patients. None of the children have undergone splenectomy so that this therapy in children cannot be evaluated. Eight adults received steroids and seven responded, although in several the response was not maintained when steroids were discontinued. Six adults underwent splenectomy and all responded, although the length of response could not be determined from the descriptions in the literature. In general, however, it appears that many patients with primary autoimmune granulocytopenia do not have major problems with infections, and treatment other than with antibiotics is not necessary. Most patients who require treatment respond well to corticosteroids or splenectomy at least temporarily, and probably should receive a trial of corticosteroids first. The recommended dose of prednisone is 1 to 2 mg/kg/day.

Intravenous immune globulin (IVIg) has been used successfully to treat autoimmune thrombocytopenia. One established mechanism of action of IVIg in autoimmune thrombocytopenia is inhibition of Fc receptor–mediated cell removal. This and other postulated mechanisms of action of IVIg are not specific for platelets.[263] Thus, IVIg has been used in a few patients with autoimmune neutropenia. Two children with primary AIN were given three and two doses of IVIg of 500 mg/kg and 450 mg/kg respectively.[264] Both achieved neutrophil counts greater than 3,000 per microliter within a few days, which gradually declined during the subsequent 2 weeks. One adult who responded to steroids, but relapsed when they were withdrawn, responded to high-dose IVIg[265] in a manner similar to patients with autoimmune thrombocytopenia. Since corticosteroids alter granulocyte and monocyte function, it may be desirable to attempt a course of IVIg before steroids in patients who require therapy because of serious infections. Additional clinical experience will be necessary to better define the value of IVIg. Two patients have received and responded to cyclophosphamide.[117,265] This therapy must be considered experimental and should be reserved for patients who have serious infections and fail to respond to the usual therapy.

Minnesota Experience with Primary AIN   During the last several years we have studied 36 patients who clinically appear to have primary autoimmune neutropenia. Twenty-two patients were male and 14 were female. The patients ranged in age from 4½ months to 7 years, with a median of 12 months. While all patients' sera had antigranulocyte activity, specificity for known granulocyte antigens was present in 17 and lacking in 19. Notably, all 17 patients who had a granulocyte antibody with known specificity had anti-NA1. The sera from all patients was tested by granulocyte agglutination, granulocyte immunofluorescence, and lymphocytotoxicity. All sera reacted by agglutination, and 34 of the 36 reacted by immunofluorescence. However, only five sera of 29 tested reacted by lymphocytotoxicity. Four of the five sera with lymphocytotoxic activity reacted weakly, and only with a few (5% to 30%) cells tested. Thus, in our experience, HLA or lymphocytotoxic reactivity is not striking in these patients. The immunoglobulin class of antibody was determined in 24 of the 36 patients. Eighteen patients had antigranulocyte activity which was IgG only, and in two patients the activity was IgM only. Four other patients had sera with a mixture of IgG and IgM activity. There was no apparent relationship between the immunoglobulin class of the antibody and the strength or character of reactivity in the different leukocyte antibody assays or the clinical course of the patient.

Natural History   Long-term follow-up reports are not available on most patients reported in the literature, so the natural history of

Table 9-4. Laboratory Aspects of Primary Autoimmune Neutropenia

Reference	Antibody Method	Antibody Specificity	WBC/μl	PMN/μl	Lymphs/μl	Eos/μl	Mono/μl	Marrow Cellularity	Marrow Description
Lalezari et al[173]	GA	NA2	9,000	990	1,029	0	1,881	Hyper	↓ PMNs
Boxer et al[19]	Opsonic	NR	NR	70	NR	NR	NR	NR	Normal myeloid maturation
	Opsonic	NR	1,000	20	780	0	200	Normal	Normal myeloid maturation
	Opsonic	NR	"Normal"	285	"Normal"	NR	NR	NR	↓ M/E ratio; ↓ PMNs
	Opsonic	NR	900	108	892	0	0	Hyper	Slight left shift
	Opsonic	NR	NR	1,000	NR	NR	NR	NR	NR
Valbonesi et al[365]	GA and GIF	NA1	1,200	120	1,068	240	84	NR	Arrest at myelocyte stage
Verheugt et al[82]	GIF	ND1	1,500	720	645	15	120	NR	↓ Myeloid; ↑ lymphs
	GIF	NA1	11,600	116	10,324	232	928	NR	Arrest at myelocyte stage
Lightsey et al[363]	Opsonic and Fab anti-Fab	NR	7,200	144	6,768	0	288	Hyper	M/E 15:1; ↓ PMNs
Cline et al[117]	GC	NR	1,500	630	840	30	0	Hyper	Arrest at promyelocyte stage
McCullough et al[29]	GA	NA1	5,000	100	3,000	5	900	Hyper	M/E 18:1; no maturation arrest
	GA	NA1	6,200	310	5,270	62	558	Hyper	M/E 12:1; arrest at band stage
Claas et al[180]	GA and GIF	NA2	NR	NR	NR	NR	NR	NR	NR
	GA and GIF	NA2	NR	NR	NR	NR	NR	NR	NR
	GA and GIF	NE1	NR	NR	NR	NR	NR	NR	NR

Reference	Method							Marrow	Marrow description
Thompson et al[233]	GA and GC	NR	9,300	90	8,100	900	200	Mod hyper	Myeloid hyperplasia; no PMNs present
Nepo et al[366]	Opsonic and phagocytic	NR	5,700	285	NR	NR	NR	Normal	M/E 5:1; ↓ PMNs
Madyastha et al[367]	GA and GIF	NA1	11,000	770	NR	NR	NR	NR	↓ PMNs
Kay et al[368]	GA	NR	6,900	207	6,420	69	207	Normal	Arrest at myelocyte stage
Blashke et al[77]	GC	NR	1,100	33	825	231	110	Normal	↓ Myeloid; arrest at myelocyte stage
Smith et al[65]	MCA	NR	4,200	1,176	2,520	420	462	Normal	Normal myeloid development
Bom-van Noorloos et al[110]	GIF*	None	8,400	300	6,900	0	1,200	NR	Arrest at myelocyte stage
	GIF	NR	15,000	<300	14,000	NR	NR	NR	Arrest at myelocyte stage
Caligaris-Cappio et al[166]	GA	NR	NR	<500	NR	NR	NR	Normal	Arrest at metamyelocyte stage
	GA	NR	NR	300	NR	NR	NR	Normal	Arrest at metamyelocyte stage
Carmel[369]	SPA	NR	900	0	846	0	54	Normal	Absence of myeloid cells
Sabbe et al[370]	GA and GC	NA2	NR	0	NR	NR	NR	NR	Arrest at myelocyte stage
	GA and GC	NE1	NR	70	NR	NR	NR	NR	Left shift
	GA and GC	NA2	NR	0	NR	NR	NR	NR	Normal
	GA, GC and GIF	NR	NR	0	NR	NR	NR	NR	Left shift
	GC	NR	NR	10	NR	NR	NR	NR	Left shift
Freed[336]	Opsonic and SPA	NR	1,500	250	NR	NR	NR	Normal	M:E 1:1; no PMNs

ABBREVIATIONS: GA = granulocyte agglutination; GC = granulocyte cytotoxicity; GIF = granulocyte immunofluorescence; MCA = microcapillary agglutination; NR = not reported; PMN = polymorphonuclear leukocytes; SPA = staph protein A.

* Patient had increased Tγ or natural killer lymphocytes.

primary autoimmune neutropenia is not well defined. Blaschke et al[77] reported one patient with what appeared to be primary autoimmune granulocytopenia, who developed Hodgkin's disease 2 years later. Apparently, most of the children recovered spontaneously in 6 to 12 months with no sequelae.[9]

The neutrophil count has now returned to normal in five of the 36 patients we have studied. The course of one of these is shown diagrammatically in Figure 9–2, which illustrates the long-term course of the disease. In these five patients, neutropenia was detected at 4½ to 16½ months of age (median 8 months). IgG granulocyte antibodies with anti-NA1 specificity were detected in each case. The titers of these antibodies, generally inversely proportional to the absolute neutrophil counts, decreased throughout their clinical course and eventually disappeared. The neutropenia resolved spontaneously in all five cases, without immunosuppressive therapy and splenectomy. The duration of the neutropenia ranged from 6½ to 35 months (median 12 months).

During the neutropenic period, these patients experienced repeated mild to moderate infections, but these were adequately managed with antibiotics and standard care. Of the 65 documented infections, the most common was otitis media followed by a variety of other infections (Table 9–5). This represented a substantial increase in infections compared to their previous history. These five patients had a median of 4.3 (range 0 to 8) infections per year before the onset of neutropenia. This increased to a median of 8 (range 5 to 12) during neutropenia, with a median of 6.7 infections

---

Figure 9–2.

Neutrophil levels relative to anti-NA1 in a patient with primary autoimmune neutropenia.

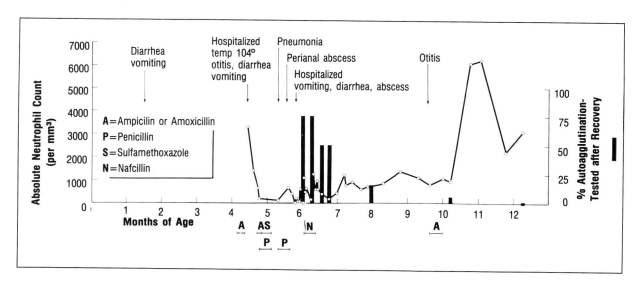

Table 9-5. **Sixty-five Infections in Five Patients with Primary Autoimmune Neutropenia**

Infections	Percentage
Otitis media	40
Skin infection	17
Upper respiratory tract	16
Gastroenteritis	9
Pharyngitis	5
Pneumonia	5
Tonsillitis	3
Perianal or perirectal abscess	1
Bronchitis	1
Croup	1
Urinary tract infection	1
Conjunctivitis	1
	100

per year requiring antibiotics. After a return of the neutrophil count to normal, the incidence of infections returned to the previously low levels (median 2.3, range 1.5 to 4.8 per year).

Following the return of a sustained normal neutrophil count, the patients were followed for 8 to 66 months (median 41 months). They were seen by their local physicians for repeated history, physical examination, and complete blood counts. Three of the patients experienced an accelerated weight gain, and there has been no evidence of other disease, particularly of autoimmune disease, during the follow-up period. Thus, it appears that, typically, infections in these patients are not life-threatening and the disease is self-limited. The routine use of corticosteroids or splenectomy does not seem indicated. Antimicrobial therapy of infectious complications is a reasonable and conservative treatment approach in uncomplicated cases. The neutropenia can be expected to resolve spontaneously in approximately 12 months, and these patients would not be expected to develop other autoimmune diseases.

Secondary Autoimmune Neutropenia

Neutropenia is a common factor in many autoimmune diseases. The mechanism for this is often not well defined and it probably varies in different situations. Some possible mechanisms include the following: (1) autoantibodies against other tissues may cross-react with granulocyte surface determinants, (2) immune complexes may be deposited on the granulocytes, (3) IgG autoantibodies may nonspecifically attach to the surface of granulocytes, and (4) complement activation may lead to deposition of complement components on granulocytes. A brief summary of the different diseases in which immune neutropenia has been reported follows.

Autoimmune Hemolytic Anemia (AIHA)   Leukopenia and thrombocytopenia are commonly seen in patients with AIHA and may represent a spectrum of autoimmune phenomena involving different cell lines.[266] One of the original and classic descriptions of immune granulocytopenia was of a patient who developed autoimmune hemolytic anemia, thrombocytopenia, and granulocytopenia after primary atypical pneumonia, presumably due to *Mycoplasma pneumoniae*.[245] The patient's plasma caused severe granulocytopenia when transfused into a normal subject, even though the leukoagglutinin was active only at 0°C.

Evans syndrome is primary thrombocytopenic purpura and hemolytic anemia occuring either simultaneously or in succession and with no underlying cause. Neutropenia, usually recurrent, occurs in 25% to 75% of these patients.[266,267] The sera of most of these patients reacts by GIF, and in one study all of the 24 patients had immunoglobulin coating their cells (positive direct GIF).[268] Absorption and elution studies suggested that the autoantibodies were specific for different blood cells. This is supported by the identification of separate autoantibodies against red blood cells and platelets in two patients with pancytopenia.[269] Corticosteroids may be transiently effective, but these patients usually become refractory to immunosuppressive therapy. Splenectomy usually results in immediate improvement, but relapse is common.[266,267]

Granulocytopenia and thrombocytopenia may also occur together in the absence of immune hemolytic anemia.[270] This also seems to be an autoimmune process, as both granulocyte and platelet antibodies have been demonstrated. The one patient reported responded well to splenectomy, with disappearance of the autoantibodies.

Systemic Lupus Erythematosus (SLE)   Granulocytopenia is commonly associated with SLE. Since many patients with SLE have circulating immune complexes,[121,165] it is possible that these might cause granulocytopenia by binding to the patient's granulocytes. Patients with SLE have increased granulocyte-associated IgG, which does not correlate with the granulocyte count, however. It appears that the increased granulocyte-associated IgG results from binding of both circulating immune complexes and granulocyte autoantibodies.[121] Granulocyte autoantibodies occur in patients with SLE.[79,271,272] Most of these antibodies have been detected with a cytotoxicity assay, but their significance is questionable because subsequent work with the method suggests that the technique was too sensitive and results may not be clinically meaningful.[24,79] The sera of 26 of 28 SLE patients tested caused granulocyte aggregation[273] similar to that seen in dialysis-induced neutropenia and adult respiratory distress syndrome. This was not correlated with circulating immune complexes, and the authors suggested that the formation of granulocyte microaggregates might have a role in the pathophysiology of SLE. A practical diagnostic test to determine the cause of granulocytopenia in patients with SLE is not presently available to aid in patient care. However, efforts to determine whether there is increased granulocyte-associated IgG are probably valuable because such patients reportedly respond well to corticosteroids.[274]

Felty's Syndrome   The exact cause of granulocytopenia of Felty's syndrome (rheumatoid arthritis, splenomegaly, and granulocytopenia) is not known, but an immunologic mechanism seems to be involved. This conclusion is based on several observations including increased granulocyte-associated IgG, presence of intracellular immunoglobulin inclusions, cryoglobulins, immune complexes, and granulocyte-specific antibodies.

Patients with Felty's syndrome have an increased amount of granulocyte-associated IgG; however, data is contradictory as to whether this correlates with the granulocyte count.[122,269,275,276] Granulocyte-associated IgG declines following splenectomy, which is correlated with the increase in granulocyte count. The increased granulocyte-associated IgG is thought to be due to granulocyte autoantibodies, or binding of immune complexes to granulocytes, or both. Patients with Felty's syndrome have higher levels of circulating immune complexes than patients with rheumatoid arthritis alone. The presence of these immune complexes correlates with granulocyte-associated IgG levels.[122] However, many patients also have increased antigranulocyte activity in their serum, so that the granulocyte-associated IgG may be due to both immune complexes and granulocyte antibodies.

The process causing neutropenia in Felty's syndrome is not clear. The antigranulocyte IgG may bind to granulocytes nonspecifically, possibly by binding to Fc receptors, then causing accelerated removal of the granulocytes from the circulation.[277] Some of the granulocyte antibodies may activate complement and lead to accelerated granulocyte removal.[168] Vincent et al[278] found excessive margination of granulocytes in patients with Felty's syndrome that, according to their calculations, could entirely account for the granulocytopenia. Joyce et al[279] proposed that the granulocytopenia of Felty's syndrome is due to many factors, the predominant one being deficient granulocyte production related to lack of a compensatory increase in bone marrow activity. This is possibly due to immune destruction of myeloid precursors.[280] Granulocyte antibodies were detected in many patients, but there was no relationship between the presence of antibodies and granulocyte survival. Thus, although immune destruction of granulocytes plays a role in patients with Felty's syndrome, the lack of compensatory increase in granulocyte production is an additional key factor. Some patients with Felty's syndrome who do not respond to splenectomy develop antibody-dependent lymphocyte-mediated granulocytotoxicity[114] so that cell-mediated immune mechanisms may also be involved.

Neutropenia is also common in patients with rheumatoid arthritis who do not have Felty's syndrome. Most of these patients have not been subjected to careful leukocyte serologic studies. In general, it appears that rheumatoid arthritis patients who are neutropenic have more extensive disease and a lower bone marrow neutrophil reserve, and are more likely to have circulating immune complexes.[281] In a detailed analysis of bone marrow morphology, patients with rheumatoid arthritis had evidence of mitotic pool depletion, suggesting that the major problem was failure of the marrow to maintain normal neutrophil levels in the peripheral blood. By contrast, two patients with Felty's syndrome had a pattern characteristic of cell destruction (increased mitotic pool and decreased segmented neutrophils), although other patients' marrows showed evidence of impaired myeloid proliferation, maturation, or release.[282]

Neutropenia has also been reported in association with Sjogren's syndrome, a collagen disease that may accompany other rheumatic diseases.[283] Serum IgG antigranulocyte binding and in vivo granulocyte kinetic studies in one patient suggested immune destruction of granulocytes.

Infectious Mononucleosis Severe granulocytopenia is a rare complication of infectious mononucleosis, occurring in approximately 0.36% of cases.[284] It usually develops 3 to 4 weeks after the onset of symptoms, lasts about a week, and spontaneously resolves. Although granulocytopenia appeared to be related to an opsonic granulocyte antibody in one case,[284] a larger study of 14 patients with EB virus infectious mononucleosis showed that 12 had granulocyte antibodies, although many were not neutropenic.[285] EB virus infection causes B-lymphocyte activation and production of IgG, IgM, and IgA. Much of this antibody activity is against antigens unrelated to EB virus. Thus, it seems likely that this general process results in some antigranulocyte activity that, for reasons not now known, causes granulocytopenia in certain patients.

Lymphatic Malignancies Malignant lymphoproliferative diseases are known to be associated with autoimmune hemolytic anemia or thrombocytopenic purpura. Recently, autoimmune granulocytopenia has been reported in association with an unusual helper T-cell leukemia in which the patient also had granulocyte autoantibodies.[286] Granulocytopenia has been reported due to autoantibodies in a patient with Hodgkin's disease.[287,288] In one patient there was an increase in serum antigranulocyte activity and granulocyte-associated IgG, both of which were inversely related to the patient's granulocyte count.[287] The patient's bone marrow was not involved with the malignancy, and similar antigranulocyte activity was not found in other patients with Hodgkin's disease. The disappearance of granulocyte antibody and return of the granulocyte count to normal after successful therapy of the patient's disease add to the evidence that this represented autoimmune granulocytopenia secondary to the lymphatic malignancy. From these reports, it seems likely that autoimmune granulocytopenia will be found increasingly in association with a variety of lymphoproliferative disorders. The association of granulocytopenia with benign T-lymphocytes will be discussed later (see section on cellular destruction of granulocytes, chapter 9).

Immune Deficiency Diseases   Granulocytopenia is a recognized complication in patients with severe hypogammaglobulinemia and infection. This rarely occurs in patients receiving immune serum globulin and, since the patients are usually infected, the granulocytopenia is often thought to be due to suppression of myelopoiesis by endotoxin. However, autoimmune granulocytopenia has been reported in two adults who were not infected and were receiving immune globulin.[289] There was a normal level of T-suppressor lymphocytes so that proliferation of lymphocytes producing autoantibody was probably not responsible for the granulocytopenia. Since both patients responded to vincristine and not to corticosteroids, it is important to recognize rapidly progressive granulocytopenia in these patients and not use steroids, which might increase the susceptibility to infection.

Thyroid Disease   Granulocytopenia occurs in relation to thyroid disease, but it is usually caused by drugs, propylthiouracil and methimazole, used to treat hyperthyroidism. Granulocytopenia usually occurs within 2 months of beginning drug therapy, is more common in older patients, and may be related to the dose of the drug.[290] It is not known whether the granulocytopenia is due to drug antibodies or toxic suppression of the bone marrow. Thus, it is possible that granulocytopenia related to thyroid disease is not even appropriately included in this discussion.

Mannosidosis   The oldest described patient with the inherited lysosomal storage disease, mannosidosis, had pancytopenia with antibodies against red blood cells, platelets, and granulocytes.[291] It was postulated that an abnormal accumulation of mannose-rich glycoproteins or oligosaccharides created neoantigens, resulting in autoantibody formation.

Scleroderma   One patient with scleroderma has been reported who developed what appeared to be autoimmune granulocytopenia.[292] Myeloid precursors were absent from the bone marrow and leukocytotoxic antibodies were present. However, it was not specified whether the antibodies were granulocyte-specific, nor whether their presence coincided with the granulocytopenia. The patient responded to corticosteroid therapy.

Drug-Related Neutropenia

In one analysis of drug-induced hematologic disorders, 18 cases of isolated granulocytopenia occurred during ten years in a group medical care population of 225,000 persons.[293] The drug most commonly involved was sulfasalazine. Granulocytopenia developed with an incidence of one in 220 patients receiving this drug and one in 422 patients who received procainamide. Although laboratory studies were not done to determine whether these cases of granulocytopenia were immune-mediated, this study provides a unique opportunity to survey the scope of drug-related granulocytopenia.

Many drugs cause granulocytopenia by a toxic effect on myelopoiesis. It also appears that some drugs cause granulocytopenia by immune destruction of mature granulocytes. In a classic experiment, Moeschlin and Wagner[6] showed that plasma from a patient who developed agranulocytosis while receiving aminopyrine caused severe neutropenia when transfused into a normal subject. The mechanism of drug-related immune granulocytopenia is probably similar to that involving red blood cells. It is usually necessary that the drug be present in the in vitro test system,[140,147,294] which suggests that there may be either (1) drug-antibody immune complex formation with binding to the granulocyte, or (2) drug acting as a hapten on the granulocyte with antibody formation against that complex. Other cases of drug-related immune granulocytopenia due to IgG non–drug-dependent autoantibodies,[140] or IgM cytotoxic antibodies,[141,151] or IgG complement-fixing antibodies,[295] have been reported. It seems likely that as test methods are improved and the capability to study drug-related granulocytopenia is more widely available, an increasing number of drugs will be implicated in immune destruction of mature granulocytes.

In the largest reported study of drug-related immune granulocytopenia, all 16 patients had opsonic antibodies against granulocytes.[140] The drugs involved were semisynthetic penicillins (nafcillin, dicloxacillin, oxacillin), procainamide, sulfafurazole, cefoxitin, propylthiouracil, methimazole, gold thiomalate, and quinidine.[104,147,148,151] Toxic effects on the bone marrow or dose-related direct cell toxicity have been thought to be the most common mechanisms involved in neutropenia associated with penicillin and its derivatives. Rouviex et al,[146] however, found B-lactamine leukoagglutinating antibodies in eight of nine patients who developed neutropenia while receiving penicillin or its derivatives. In a review of neutropenia associated with benzylpenicillin (penicillin G), Snavely et al[296] point out that this almost always occurs when large doses are given intravenously for about 3 weeks. The neutropenia usually lasts about 7 days after the drug is discontinued. However, Rouviex et al[146] noted that drug-related neutropenia occurred in some patients receiving oral therapy with doses as low as 40 mg per kg per 24 hr.

Granulocytopenia has resulted from phenytoin (Dilantin), but it is not clear whether this was due to immune destruction of mature granulocytes or suppression of myelopoiesis.[297] Granulocytotoxic autoantibodies occur in granulocytopenic patients receiving levamisol.[149] The antibodies seem to be directed against mature granulocytes only, and their presence coincides with granulocytopenia. Thus, this appears to be one of the clearer examples of drug-related immune granulocytopenia. Granulocytopenia is a well-known complication of tricyclic antidepressant drugs, although the causative mechanism is not known. A recent report of granulocytopenia in association with the tricyclic antidepressant maprotiline is of interest because the patient's bone marrow showed myeloid hyperplasia with absence of mature granulocytes.[298] This is similar to the bone marrow findings in many patients with alloimmune neonatal neutropenia and autoimmune granulocytopenia where the pathophysiologic mechanism is clearly due to granulocyte-specific antibodies. However, it appears that granulocytopenia due to the tricyclic imipramine is due to bone marrow toxicity rather than immune destruction of mature granulocytes.[299]

The antithyroid drugs propylthiouracil, methimazole, and carbimazole share a thioamide group, which has been proposed as the antigenic determinant causing immune neutropenia from these drugs.[300] This immune neutropenia may not be due merely to antibody. In five of six patients who experienced neutropenia due to these drugs, there was significant in vitro lymphocyte transformation in response to the drugs. Since patients with thyroiditis who are receiving these drugs have an immunologic abnormality, the immune neutropenia may represent another manifestation of altered immunity in these patients.[300]

Studies of the kinetics of drug-associated granulocyte antibodies have shown that, although the initial antibody titer or strength of reactivity may be high, antibody activity quickly declines after cessation of drug and is usually absent upon return of normal granulocyte counts.[140,141,146,149-151] This was especially emphasized in the study of patients with neutropenia due to B-lactamine antibodies.[146] The antibody titers were low, and in one case antibody activity was gone 5 days after discontinuation of drug. In their studies, serum obtained within 1 day after the drug was stopped did not require the addition of drug to demonstrate drug antibody activity. However, when using serum from day 2 or 3, agglutination was more easily detected with drug addition.

Hence, for successful detection of drug-induced granulocyte antibodies, it is important to get patient serum samples during the nadir of the patient's granulocytopenia, soon after the drug has been discontinued and after the patient's granulocyte count has returned to normal. Conclusive evidence for the presence of a drug-associated autoimmune mechanism is obtained by testing the patient's granulocytes upon recovery with the patient's serum (with and without the addition of drug) obtained during various phases of the disease course.

Role of Immune Complexes in Neutropenia

Immune complexes have been reported in a high proportion of patients with chronic idiopathic granulocytopenia.[166,167] It has been suggested that these are a causative factor in the granulocytopenia, either through complement activation or increased removal of granulocytes by the reticuloendothelial system. The antigen involved and origin of the immune complexes in these patients is not known. Sera from two patients with idiopathic granulocytopenia and circulating immune complexes, when injected into rabbits, caused pulmonary sequestration of granulocytes.[166] However, since these patients' sera also had leukoagglutinating activity, it is difficult to distinguish the role of the immune complexes. Clinical follow-up of one group of patients supported the pathologic role of immune complexes using the following reasoning: Patients with immune complexes had a bone marrow myeloid maturation arrest at the metamyelocyte stage, whereas patients without immune complexes had a maturation arrest involving less mature cells. The former group had a benign clinical course consistent with peripheral destruction of granulocytes. The latter group had a more severe course including development of anemia and/or thrombocytopenia, myelogenous leukemia, and death due to widespread infection, suggesting that an abnormal bone marrow was the fundamental problem.

Patients with systemic lupus erythematosus (SLE) or Felty's syndrome have high levels of circulating immune complexes and increased granulocyte-associated IgG.[121,122] In one study, the level of granulocyte-associated IgG was related to the level of circulating immune complexes.[121] However, it appears that the granulocyte-associated IgG results both from binding of circulating immune complexes to granulocytes and also from serum antigranulocyte activity.

We have investigated the relationship among immune complexes, granulocyte antibodies, and autoimmune neutropenia (AIN). Sera from neutropenic patients were tested for granulocyte antibodies using the GA and GIF assays and were tested for immune complexes using an iodine 125-C1q binding test. Of the patients used in the test, 29 were diagnosed with primary AIN, seven with a neutropenia of unknown etiology, six with Felty's syndrome, five with SLE, two with alloimmune neonatal neutropenia, one with autoimmune thrombocytopenic purpura (ATP), and one with Crohn's disease. Although the 29 juvenile patients with primary AIN all had GA and/or GIF antibodies, only two had immune complexes detected in their serum (Table 9–6). Sixteen of the 29 patients had antibodies specific for known granulocyte antigens (15 NA1, 1 NA2),

Table 9–6.   **Circulating Immune Complexes and Granulocyte Antibodies in Patients with Primary and Secondary AIN**

Primary AIN Patients

		GA +	GA −	GIF +	GIF −	Total
C1q-binding	+	2	0	2	0	2
	−	27	0	26	1	27
Total		29	0	28	1	

Other Patients
6 Felty's syndrome
5 SLE
7 Idiopathic neutropenia
1 Crohn's disease
2 Alloimmune neonatal neutropenia
1 ATP

		GA +	GA −	GIF +	GIF −	Total
C1q-binding	+	5[a]	0	4[b]	1[c]	5
	−	10	7	15	2	17
Total		15	7	19	3	

NOTES: Immune complexes were measured by C1q-binding; granulocyte antibodies were measured by granulocyte agglutination (GA) and granulocyte immunofluorescence (GIF).
[a]4 Felty's, 1 SLE.
[b]Felty's.
[c]SLE.

but those were not associated with the presence of immune complexes. In the remaining patient studies, immune complexes and antibodies were both detected in four of the six Felty's patients and in the one SLE patient. Thus, our studies do not indicate a major role for immune complexes in AIN; however, this remains an interesting possibility. Although circulating immune complexes may play a role in granulocyte destruction, many related issues are not understood, including the following: (1) whether immune complexes alone cause granulocytopenia, (2) whether granulocyte auto-antibodies are also involved, (3) why immune complexes might cause only granulocytopenia since there are many other possible target tissues, and (4) why many patients with circulating immune complexes are not granulocytopenic.

Cellular Destruction of Granulocytes

The mechanisms of immune destruction of granulocytes predominantly involve the interaction of antibody-coated granulocytes with phagocytic cells. Although much remains to be learned about the kind of leukocyte antibodies involved, their optimum method of detection, and the possible value of cell-associated IgG measurements, even less is known about the role of cellular immune mechanisms in the etiology of granulocytopenia. T-lymphocytes are known to regulate a variety of B-lymphocyte and T-lymphocyte functions and to have an effect in many other tissue functions. T-lymphocytes are important regulators of hematopoiesis. Thus, cellular functions might be involved in neutropenia in several ways including (1) suppression of hematopoiesis; and (2) altered regulation of B-cell function, allowing production of antibodies against myeloid precursors or mature granulocytes.

Antibody-Dependent Lymphocyte-Mediated Granulocytotoxicity (ADLG)

ADLG is the situation most similar to a purely humoral cell destruction mechanism. Logue et al[109] reported that two patients who apparently had autoimmune granulocytopenia (with SLE and rheumatoid arthritis) had ADLG activity. Such activity was postulated to be the cause of the granulocytopenia because it was not found with serum or lymphocytes alone. However, some granulocytopenic patients were identified who had increased granulocyte-associated IgG without ADLG activity. After splenectomy, some patients with Felty's syndrome developed ADLG activity that correlated with persistent granulocytopenia. Thus, this cellular immune mechanism may be responsible for the persistent granulocytopenia in these patients who are unresponsive to splenectomy.[114]

T-Cell Involvement

A number of patients with T-lymphocytosis and neutropenia have been reported.[116,301–307] Bom-van Noorloos et al[110] described two patients with chronic granulocytopenia and absolute lymphocytosis due to increased numbers of T-lymphocytes with IgG receptors. These IgG receptor–bearing T-lymphocytes had antibody-dependent lymphocytotoxicity but did not have natural killer activity.

In a larger study of 15 leukopenic patients by van der Veen et al,[133] there were four patients with a high T4/T8 ratio and nine patients with a low T4/T8 ratio. The high ratio was due to a decrease in T8 (suppressor) cells, while the low ratio was usually due to a decrease in T4 (helper) cells, except for two patients who had an increase in T8 cells. These last two patients were similar to those reported by Bom-van Noorloos et al,[110] who had a syndrome of T-lymphocytosis and neutropenia. In general, the T4/T8 ratios did not correlate with the presence of granulocyte antibodies, the neutrophil count, or bone marrow morphology.

Usually these patients with an expanded T-lymphocyte population have an increased number of IgG receptor–bearing lymphocytes, (ie, suppressor cells or killer cells or natural killer cells)[302], which are commonly referred to as Tγ cells. In most patients reported, the Tγ-cells react with OKT8, suggesting that they are suppressor cells, although in several patients the cells were functionally abnormal since they did not exhibit suppressor activity.[301,302,304,307] The neutropenia in these patients seems to be due to a humoral immune mechanism because there is increased granulocyte-associated IgG and a shortened granulocyte intravascular survival.[305] It seems likely that the neutropenia in these patients is due to granulocyte autoantibodies resulting from abnormal T-cell regulation.[305] It has been suggested that Tγ-lymphocytosis occurs more often than expected in patients with chronic idiopathic neutropenia,[306] and thus T-lymphocyte marker studies may be helpful in identifying patients who can be expected to have a benign clinical course instead of a malignant T-cell neoplasm. The syndrome can now be characterized as chronic and benign since some patients have shown no progression of their disease over 20 years. The patients have recurrent bacterial infections primarily of the skin and oropharynx, but the infections are not usually severe. Since these patients do not have progressive disease, they should be distinguished from those with T-cell chronic lymphocytic leukemia in order to avoid unnecessary therapy.

Evaluation of Neutropenia

Diagnosis of Neutropenia

Neutropenia, defined as an absolute neutrophil count of less than 1500 cells per microliter,[308] can occur at any age and has many causes. Neutropenia may be associated with other cytopenias or may present as an isolated finding. The causes of neutropenia can be divided into three general categories: (1) decreased or absent production, (2) accelerated destruction, and (3) abnormal distribution.[309] These three categories can be further subdivided as shown in Table 9–1.

The clinical significance of neutropenia is an increased risk of infection. Infection is most often superficial and caused by gram-positive cocci. Gram-negative organisms, fungi, viruses, and opportunistic organisms can also cause infections in these patients at any site. With absolute neutrophil counts of 1,000 to 1,500 per microliter the risk of infection is not increased.[261] If the absolute neutrophil count is 500 to 1,000 per microliter, the risk of infection is slightly increased. Below 500 per microliter serious infections frequently occur, particularly when this degree of neutropenia is present for more than a few days[261]. Thus, patients with an absolute neutrophil count below 1,000 per microliter should be evaluated to determine the cause of neutropenia. To establish the pattern and chronicity of the neutropenia, serial white blood cell counts with differential counts should be obtained twice weekly for 6 to 8 weeks.[261]

Clinical History and Physical Examination Once it has been established that a patient is neutropenic, the nature of the neutropenic disorder can be more clearly defined.

A careful history should be taken to determine what, if any, symptoms are associated with neutropenia. This should encompass the health of family members as well as of the patient, as some neutropenias appear to be familial.[310-313] Since infectious diseases may cause neutropenia, a history suggesting any of these is significant. Such diseases have been discussed by Murdoch and Smith[314] and are listed in Table 9–7. However, it is often not possible to exclude neutropenia prior to such an illness, particularly if there are no associated symptoms. A thorough history of any drugs currently or previously taken should be obtained since many drugs have been associated with neutropenia[140,315,316] (Table 9–8).

The signs and symptoms suggesting cyclic neutropenia include regularly recurrent fever, malaise, aphthous oral ulcers, skin infections, and cervical adenopathy. When these are present, white blood cell counts (WBC) and differentials every three days are recommended[317] to establish the cycling time and the neutrophil

---

Table 9–7.   *Infectious Diseases Possibly Associated with Neutropenia*

Measles	Syphilis
Rubella	Miliary tuberculosis
Influenza and parainfluenza	Typhus and scrub typhus
Infectious mononucleosis	Psittacosis
Hepatitis B	Histoplasmosis
Aseptic meningitis	Malaria
Typhoid and paratyphoid fever	Kala-azar
Brucellosis	Trypanosomiasis

Table 9–8.   *Drugs Associated with Neutropenia*

Penicillin and semisynthetic derivatives	Anticonvulsants
Cephalothins	Antithyroid drugs
Sulfonamides	Cardiac antiarrhythmic drugs
Aminopyrine derivatives	Diuretics
Nonsteroidal anti-inflammatory agents	Antipsychotic and antianxiety drugs
Antihistamines including cimetidine	Oral hypoglycemic agents
Antimalarials	

count when the WBC reaches its peak. Because the cycle remains fairly constant in these patients,[311,317] prediction of the WBC nadir may permit precautions to prevent infections. For example, dental procedures could be avoided during the period of neutropenia.

Neutropenia may also be associated with other noninfectious diseases, such as systemic lupus erythematosus (SLE), Felty's syndrome, congestive splenomegaly,[318] Gaucher's disease,[319], sarcoidosis, malignancy with marrow infiltration, leukemia, aplastic anemia, dysgammaglobulinemia,[312,320] Chediak-Higashi syndrome,[321] lazy leukocyte syndrome,[322] copper deficiency,[323,324] and anorexia nervosa.[325,326] These must be excluded before a diagnosis of primary neutropenia can be made.

Laboratory Studies

Complete Blood Counts Once it has been established that a patient is neutropenic, the laboratory investigation may include a variety of different tests but should to some extent be determined by the severity of the disease. An algorithm depicting an approach to evaluating the neutropenic patient is shown in Figure 9–3. Along with the history and physical examination, a repeat complete blood count (CBC) with differential and a platelet count should be performed. A CBC with decreased numbers of erythrocytes and/or platelets, in addition to granulocytopenia, suggests a process involving the entire hematopoietic system such as leukemia, aplastic or hypoplastic anemia, or a myelodysplastic disorder. A patient who is consistently neutropenic but manifests no signs or symptoms, or a patient with cyclic neutropenia, will generally require no further workup.

Testing for Drug-Related Neutropenia If a drug is thought to be responsible for neutropenia, two possible steps can be taken. If the drug can be discontinued and the patient's neutrophil count returns to normal, the drug may be presumed to be the causative agent, and then no further workup is required. However, if discontinuing the drug would compromise patient treatment or does not result in resolution of neutropenia, a bone marrow aspirate/biopsy can be performed. An alternative approach is to test for granulocyte antibody activity with and without the presence of the drug in vitro. This has the advantage of eliminating the need for a bone marrow examination if a drug-dependent antibody is detected. However, the methods for detecting drug-associated granulocyte antibodies have not been as thoroughly developed as for drug-associated erythrocyte destruction. Another disadvantage is that some drug-associated neutropenias are caused by drug interactions at the level of the hematopoietic stem cell (see below). These may not be detected with conventional drug-antibody testing.

Figure 9-3.

Suggested protocol showing the role of granulocyte antibody testing in the evaluation of the neutropenic patient.

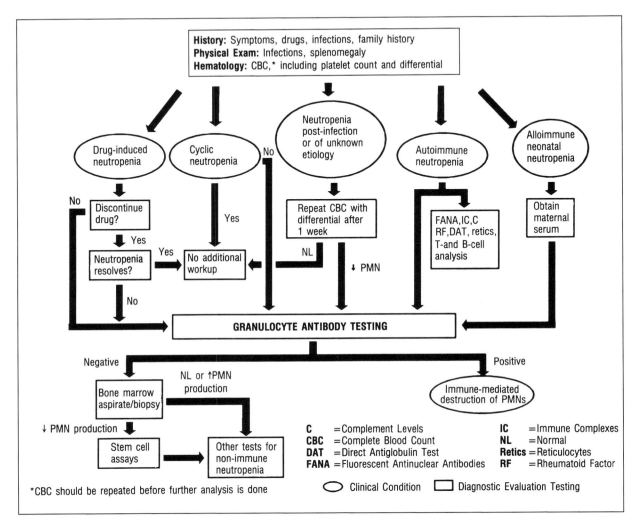

Granulocyte Antibody Detection Testing for granulocyte antibodies can be done either before or after the bone marrow examination. However, the finding of granulocyte antibodies along with clinical and laboratory findings consistent with autoimmune neutropenia can eliminate the need for bone marrow studies, especially in patients with mild to moderate symptoms. This approach has the advantages that granulocyte antibody testing is not an invasive procedure and is relatively inexpensive. Testing for granulocyte antibodies *after* bone marrow examination is indicated when the bone marrow demonstrates normal or increased cellularity with diminished or absent late granulocyte forms.

Bone Marrow Studies   The bone marrow aspirate and biopsy are useful in evaluating the cause of neutropenia. Although the marrow cellularity and myeloid-to-erythroid ratio vary somewhat by age,[327] the cellularity of normal marrow should be at least 50% and the myeloid-to-erythroid ratio about 3:1. Approximately 60% of the cells will be of the granulocytic series, 20% of the erythroid series, and 15% to 20% will be lymphocytes. Any of the disorders listed in Table 9–1 which are due to decreased granulopoiesis will have a marrow with reduced numbers of all granulocyte precursors. Neutropenia secondary to increased peripheral neutrophil destruction usually has a marrow showing normal or increased numbers of granulocyte precursors, with band and segmented forms virtually absent from the marrow. Although this pattern has been referred to as "maturation arrest,"[310,328] this is a misnomer in this case since mature forms are absent, not because of a production defect, but because of increased destruction of mature granulocytes.

Stem Cell Cultures   An extension of the bone marrow examination is a hematopoietic stem cell assay, which is becoming more widely available. Two types may be applied to the evaluation of the neutropenic patient when the marrow examination demonstrates decreased production. A sample of the patient's bone marrow can be assayed to determine the number of committed granulocyte and monocyte precursors (CFU-C or CFU-GM); a decreased number of precursors suggests a production defect. A second assay for colony-stimulating activity (CSA) can be performed using patient serum and normal bone marrow to test for cytotoxicity or inhibition of normal marrow growth in culture. If the neutropenia is thought to be drug-related, the CFU-C and CSA assays can be performed with and without the presence of the suspected drug. Unfortunately, these tests have not been well standardized for these situations. The CFU-C may be reported as an absolute number of colonies or as the number per milliliter of marrow, or based on the number of mononuclear cells tested. However, the number of mononuclear cells and total volume of marrow obtained will depend on the technique of the person obtaining the marrow. A markedly decreased number of precursors should be detected by the assay, but lesser reductions may not be identified due to the variability of the test. When CFU-C and CSA assays are performed to detect inhibition of marrow growth, either by serum from the neutropenic patient or by a drug, the results are easier to quantitate since the laboratory can report the percent inhibition compared with a normal control. Studies have demonstrated inhibition of marrow growth in the presence of trimethoprim-sulfamethoxazole,[329] cimetidine,[330] cephalosporins and semisynthetic penicillins,[331–332] quinidine,[333] procainamide,[334] and ibuprofen.[335]

Summary of Evaluation

The systematic approach described here determines whether neutropenia is present, whether this is a stable or cyclic neutropenia, and whether other blood cell lines are involved. A careful clinical history and related laboratory studies are done to identify diseases or drugs which may be causing the neutropenia. Properly timed studies of the patient's serum for granulocyte antibodies and a bone marrow analysis should make it possible to establish the diagnosis with considerable certainty. This is of practical value since the growing amount of information available about immune neutropenias makes it possible to develop a knowledgeable plan for patient care as summarized briefly below.

General Approaches to Management of Immune Neutropenia

Therapy of the neutropenia should be based on the severity of signs and symptoms related to neutropenia and its underlying cause. Infection should be treated symptomatically, and drugs that may induce or accentuate neutropenia should be avoided. If a drug is implicated as the cause of neutropenia, it should be discontinued when possible. Bone marrow examination, drug-antibody studies, and hematopoietic stem cell assays may be beneficial to exclude drug-associated neutropenia. Immune-mediated neutropenias with granulocyte antibodies have been treated with splenectomy,[148,309] steroids,[148,309] intravenous immunoglobulin,[309,336] and other immunosuppressive drugs[117] with variable success in primary autoimmune neutropenia. The neutropenic children we have followed through resolution (see Primary Autoimmune Neutropenia, above) were usually treated only with antibiotics during their episodes of infection. Alloimmune neonatal neutropenia generally requires no therapy other than antibiotics for infections, although whole blood or plasma exchange and granulocyte transfusions have been suggested as a possible treatment for life-threatening infections.[260] Patients with SLE demonstrate correction of neutropenia when treated with either steroids alone or steroids and immunosuppressive agents.[108,274] Neutropenia with Felty's syndrome may respond to splenectomy,[276] administration of gold salts,[337] penicillamine,[338] testosterone,[339] or lithium.[340] Plasma exchange may be beneficial in patients with autoimmune neutropenia and granulocyte antibodies. Although no case reports to document this have appeared in the literature, plasma exchange has proved effective in antibody-mediated pure red blood cell aplasia,[341] aplastic anemia,[342] and autoimmune thrombocytopenic purpura.[343,344] These diseases are thought to occur via a mechanism similar to autoimmune neutropenia, so this could be considered in extreme circumstances.

Chapter 10

Granulocyte Survival and Localization In Vivo

Granulocyte Production and Life Span

Granulocytes are produced in the bone marrow and released into the circulation (intravascular space) where they have a half-life of 5 to 7 hours.[345] This short life span in the circulation is primarily because, in contrast to the red blood cells and platelets, the major functions of granulocytes occur in the tissues. Thus, the circulation is only a transient phase to enable the granulocyte to move from the site of production to the site of function. The factors that control this egress from the circulation are not well understood, but it appears that the cells leave randomly, without regard to age. Kinetics studies suggest that granulocytes have an additional life span in the tissues of approximately 4 to 5 days,[346] and it is during this time that the cell carries out its biologic functions. The normal mechanism of granulocyte senescence and removal in tissues is not well known. Granulocytes either die in the tissues or are lost through the surface of mucous membranes that have external contact. This means granulocytes are shed and can be found in saliva, urine, stool, and tracheal bronchial secretions.[345,346,347]

Much of the information about granulocyte production rates, body distribution pools, and intravascular kinetics has been obtained from in vivo studies of granulocytes radiolabeled in vitro with $DF^{32}p$ or chromium 51. However, $DF^{32}p$ has not been commercially available for several years and chromium 51 gives variable results because of elution and indiscriminate labeling of leukocytes, platelets, and red blood cells. External body imaging is not possible with $DF^{32}p$ and is not effective with chromium 51 because of radiation dose limitations. In order to better study immunologic destruction of granulocytes and to determine the effect in vivo of leukocyte antibodies, a technique using the radioisotope indium 111 was adopted.

Methods for the In Vivo Study of Granulocytes

Indium 111–Labeled Granulocytes

Indium 111 is an efficient label for leukocytes.[348–350] It has a half-life of 67 hours and emits gamma photons of high energy, making indium 111 ideal for external body imaging.[351] Thus, it is possible to determine the intravascular circulation of indium 111–labeled granulocytes and also observe their tissue localization by external scintillation imaging.

Indium forms a saturated complex with oxine (8-hydroxyquin-oline). The complex is neutral and lipid-soluble, which allows rapid diffusion across the granulocyte membrane. Because the indium-oxine complex has a low stability, the indium then dissociates from oxine and binds to various cytoplasmic components.[350] Indium-oxine in the concentrations used in our technique is nontoxic to the cell, and the radioisotope appears to be firmly bound to the cell since no elution of the label was demonstrated in vitro.[349,352] When plasma is present, the indium 111 dissociates from oxine and binds to transferrin, preventing leukocyte labeling. Thus, this work must be done in a plasma-free system.

The injected radioactivity (indium) is either firmly contained in the granulocytes or free in the supernatant.[350] Therefore, manipulation of post transfusion blood samples is minimal, requiring only the determination of whole-blood and plasma radioactivity. Granulocyte-associated radioactivity can be determined by subtracting plasma radioactivity from whole-blood radioactivity at each sampling time. Results are reported as counts per minute of cell-associated radioactivity per milliliter of whole blood. This is simpler than methods requiring isolation of labeled granulocytes from post-transfusion blood samples and expression of radioactivity as the number of cells isolated or milligrams of leukocyte nitrogen.

Skin Window Technique

We have modified a little-known skin window technique to evaluate the ability of granulocytes to migrate in vivo. Three 8-mm-diameter blisters are formed on the volar surface of the forearm by gentle heat and suction.[353] The blister roofs are removed aseptically and a Lucite chamber secured in place over each lesion. One milliliter of autologous serum in each chamber serves as the chemoattractant for the subsequently intravenously injected indium 111–labeled granulocytes. The chambers are left in place for 24 hours, after which the contents are removed and the number of indium 111 granulocytes in the chamber determined. Thus, the migration of the injected test cells into this skin window can be calculated.

This skin window method is quite reproducible, giving a mean of 52×10^6 cells per chamber (range 37.3 to 80.7×10^6) and a mean of 13,466 indium 111 granulocytes per chamber (range 4,696 to 38,964) in normal subjects.[352] It is not uncomfortable for the subject and gives a consistent area of exposed dermis without bleeding. The lesions remain hyperpigmented for several weeks, but none of the 34 subjects we have studied thus far has experienced scarring. This is an excellent method for determining in vivo migration of granulocytes in uninfected subjects. We have used it to study the effect of antibodies and the effect of preservation on granulocyte migration in vivo.

Granulocyte Kinetics in Normal Subjects Using Indium 111

We have determined the intravascular survival of autologous granulocytes labeled with indium 111 in many normal subjects during the last 5 years. The initial studies developing the method were done in ten subjects (Table 10–1). Curves plotted on semilog graphs showed an initial equilibration period followed by a period of linear decrease in radioactivity. In eight out of ten subjects the maximum level of radioactivity in the circulation did not occur until 30 minutes to 2 hours after injection. The mean maximum recovery of the injected indium 111 in the circulation was 30% ± 6%. The mean half-life ($t\frac{1}{2}$) measured over the most linear portion of the curve was 5.0 ± 1.6 hours. This level of recovery is somewhat lower than that reported using other isotopes. For example, using DF[32]p-labeled granulocytes, recoveries in normal subjects have been reported to range from 26% to 81%,[349] and using chromium 51–labeled leukocytes to range from 10% to 126%.[352] On the basis of

Table 10–1.   **Kinetics of Indium 111-Oxine-Labeled Granulocytes**

Subject	Number of Granulocytes Injected ($\times 10^7$)	Radioactivity (μCi)	Labeling of Granulocytes (%)	Intravascular Recovery (%)	Time of Maximum Recovery (min)	Intravascular [$t\frac{1}{2}$ (hr)]
1	2	100	73*	29	30	5.0
2	16	280	60*	41	10	8.5
3	5	280	46*	35	120	5.5
4	7	270	80	32	120	3.8
5	8	130	90	28	10	5.7
6	17	190	91	34	60	4.1
7	12	80	86	23	120	6.0
8	9	290	92	22	60	3.4
9	12	160	94	26	60	4.6
10	23	250	90	30	120	3.2
Mean (standard deviation)	11	200	89	30±5.9	NA	5.0±1.6

ABBREVIATIONS: NA=not applicable.
*Lower degree of tagging due to albumin in suspending media.

generally established data acquired with $DF^{32}p$, one would expect 40% to 50% of the transfused granulocytes to be recovered in the circulation. Because our indium-labeling procedure requires manipulation of the blood prior to transfusion, it is possible that the lower recovery is a result of irreversible damage to some cells during preparation and their immediate removal from the circulation following injection. The in vitro function assays we and others used were unable to detect the abnormal properties that might have resulted in this immediate removal of granulocytes.[349,352,354]

The granulocyte kinetics curve shows an initial phase of equilibration of up to 2 hours before the maximum intravascular recovery is reached. A similar delay of 1 to 2 hours before achieving maximum recovery has been reported by Price and Dale.[294] An increase of peripheral blood radioactivity 1 hour after transfusion is apparent in a granulocyte kinetics curve from early neutrophil kinetic studies.[355] This initial delay may represent a time in which mildly damaged cells undergo reparation in vivo before entering the circulation. We and others[351,356] have observed an initial uptake of indium activity in the lungs that disappears within the first few hours following injection. Release of granulocytes from the lungs into the circulation could account for the observed increase in circulating radioactivity during the initial 1 to 2 hours postinjection. The second phase of the granulocyte curve is a linear decrease in radioactivity that represents the disappearance of granulocytes from the circulation. In our studies the mean t½ of this phase of 5.0 hours agrees fairly well with the t½ of 5 to 7 hours reported from previous studies using $DF^{32}p$.

Indium 111 Granulocyte Localization in Normal Subjects and Patients with Inflammation

Normal Subjects

We have performed body imaging at different intervals for up to 24 hours after injection of indium 111–labeled granulocytes. As also shown by others,[351,357] during the first 1 to 2 hours after injection some lung activity was evident, but this was cleared and there was no evidence of radioactivity in the lungs by 4 hours in all normal subjects who received autologous indium 111–labeled granulocytes (Figure 10–1). The granulocytes are seen only in the liver and spleen, although occasionally some subjects show very slight uptake in the bone marrow of the pelvis and spine at 24 hours (Figure 10–2). The radioactivity in the liver and spleen reached a plateau within the first 75 minutes after injection and remained fairly constant during the following 24 hours (Table 10–2). At 24 hours after injection, approximately 27% of the administered radioactivity was in the liver and 25% in the spleen.

Figure 10–1.

Time sequence of localization of indium 111 granulocytes after injection. (A) During injection showing some indium 111 granulocytes in the right ventricle and some in the right subclavian vein, (B) indium 111 granulocytes in the lung one minute after injection, (C) some indium 111 granulocytes in the lung and most in liver and spleen 30 minutes after injection, (D) indium 111 granulocytes cleared from the lungs and in the liver and spleen 90 minutes after injection.

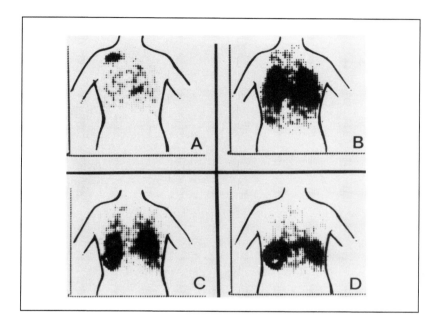

Patients with Inflammation

Indium 111 granulocytes localize at sites of inflammation.[351,356–360] Because normal uptake of radioactivity after 4 hours occurs only in the liver and spleen, the localization of indium 111–labeled granulocytes in other sites is a valuable technique for the diagnosis of inflammation or abscess. There are so many reports of the clinical use of indium 111 granulocytes that it would not be feasible to provide a comprehensive review here. The following comments focus on our experience.

Asher et al[359] found that indium 111 granulocytes had an accuracy rate of 85% in identifying intra-abdominal infection in postoperative patients. There were a 3% false positive, 9% false negative, and 3% equivocal rate. Other studies report the effectiveness of indium 111 granulocytes in localizing inflammation in the knee (rheumatoid arthritis), at sites of intramuscular injection,[356] and

Figure 10–2.

Normal body scan showing indium 111 granulocytes in the liver and spleen but no localization elsewhere in the body.

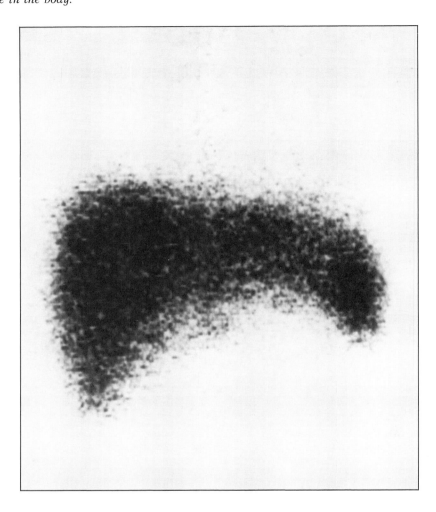

in sinus, mandible, gingiva, toe, uterus, and rectum.[357] The latter report emphasized rapid diagnostic value since the inflammatory lesions often could be visualized within 30 minutes after injection of labeled granulocytes. It appears that indium 111 granulocytes may be helpful in recognizing rejection of a transplanted kidney[358] and in identifying inflammation due to localized or systemic fungal infections.[361]

During a 2-year period, indium 111 granulocytes were used at our hospital in 411 subjects who had clinically suspected occult inflammation.[362] The study included 354 adults and 51 pediatric patients, with ages ranging from 10 months to 86 years. Leukocytes

Table 10–2.   *Percentage of Uptake of Indium 111 Radioactivity in Various Tissues After Injection of Indium 111 Granulocytes*

	4 Hours			20 Hours		
	Mean	±S.D.	Range	Mean	±S.D.	Range
Spleen	29	±9.0	(23-45)	25	±6.3	(19-34)
Liver	21	±4.8	(13-35)	27	±5.9	(20-37)
Lungs	8	±3.0	(5-13)	8	±4.2	(4-14)
Bone/Bone Marrow	5	±2.3	(3-8)	6	±3.3	(2-10)

Time After Injection (spanning both 4 Hours and 20 Hours)

ABBREVIATION: SD = standard deviation.
NOTE: Six normal subjects were studied.

for labeling were obtained from the patients or, in leukopenic patients (22 cases), from ABO-compatible normal donors. There was localization of indium 111 granulocytes at a confirmed site of inflammation in 132 of 152 cases, representing a test sensitivity of 87%. The calculated test specificity was 92% for an overall diagnostic accuracy of approximately 90%. Homologous normal donor leukocytes were equally as effective as autologous cells in detecting localized inflammation. The noninvasive nature of this test, its high accuracy rate, and its ease of administration make it a valuable addition to diagnosis of occult inflammation.

Effect of Leukocyte Antibodies on the Fate of Granulocytes In Vivo

Many methods are available to detect leukocyte antibodies;[255] however, the relationship of these tests to immune destruction of granulocytes and, thus, to different clinical situations is not clear. Since complex technical aspects of the assays limit most laboratories to routine performance of only one or two, few studies have compared the value of different antibody methods in various clinical situations involving immune destruction.

Because there has not been a method available to study the in vivo fate of transfused granulocytes, the effect of antibodies on them could not be well defined. The methods described above involving the isotope indium 111 make it possible to study the intravascular circulation and tissue localization of granulocytes in the presence of various kinds of leukocyte antibodies. We have determined the in vivo fate of indium 111 granulocytes in 93 different studies. Sera from patients were tested by granulocyte agglutination (GA), granulocytotoxicity (GC), granulocyte immunofluorescence (GIF), lymphocytotoxicity (LC), and antibody-dependent lymphocyte-mediated granulocytotoxicity (ADLG). Granulocytes from donors incompatible in one or more of these assays were labeled with indium 111 and injected. Then the intravascular recovery and survival of the indium 111 granulocytes were determined in a study of 53 subjects (Table 10–3). Antibodies detected by granulocyte agglutination were associated with a significant reduction in recovery (6.7% v 30.8% in controls; p < .001) and t½ (0.3 hours v 5.6 hours in controls; p = .002). When all possible combinations of serum reactivity were considered, reactivity in the GA plus GIF assays had the best correlation with decreased recovery (R^2 = .49; p < .001) and t½ (R^2 = .73; p < .001). When the relationship between the strength of antibody reactivity and the recovery and t½ was analyzed, LC plus GIF reactivity best correlated with decreased recovery (R^2 = .62; p = .001).

Because of the general availability of the HLA (LC) testing, the role of LC reactivity was investigated in other ways. There was a strong relationship between sera highly reactive by LC (> 60% panel cells positive) and those reactive by GIF. These highly reactive sera were more likely to be associated with abnormal intravascular granulocyte kinetics (ie, reduced recovery and t½) (Table 10–4).

The influence of HLA antigen mismatches was also studied in two different ways. The intravascular recovery and survival of in-

Table 10–3. **Effects of Leukocyte Antibodies on Intravascular Recovery and Half-Life (t½) of Indium 111 Granulocytes**

Antibody	Nonneutropenic			Neutropenic		
	n	Recovery %	t½ (hr)	n	Recovery (%)	t½ (hr)
None	9	30.8	5.6	9	10.7	5.4
GA	1	6.7[b]	0.3[b]	2	14.5	0.5[b]
GA + others	4	9.7[b]	0.3[b]	3	5.2	0.2[b]
GC	2	27.9	3.5	6	17.3	4.7
GC + others[a]	0	NA	NA	7	9.7	3.9
LC	0	NA	NA	1	25.0	ND
LC + others[a]	2	24.5	3.0	6	9.3	3.6
GIF	0	NA	NA	1	16.4	9.6
GIF + others[a]	1	16.2[b]	1.4[b]	6	9.3	3.6
ADLG	1	23.6	2.9	4	17.1	4.5
ADLG + others[a]	1	32.8	4.0	3	7.4	2.2

ABBREVIATIONS: NA=not applicable; ND=No data.

NOTES: Fifty-three patients were studied. The total shown is more than 53 because studies involving multiple antibodies were grouped in different combinations.

[a]Excludes GA antibodies.

[b]p < .01. p values are from comparison of the particular group with patients who had no antibodies.

Table 10–4. **Influence of LC Reactivity on the Reactivity in Other Tests and on Reduced Granulocyte Recovery (R) and Half-Life (t½)**

Percentage LC Panel Donors Reactive	n	Percentage Sera reactive by				Reduced R and t½
		GA	GIF	GC	ADLG	
<60	13	8	23	38	31	1 of 4
>60	15	33	93	47	20	6 of 8

Table 10–5. **Influence of Donor-Recipient Mismatching for Selected HLA Antigens on the Recovery and Half-Life (t½) of Indium 111 Granulocytes**

HLA Antigen	Recovery				t½			
	Matched Donor-Recipient		Mismatched Donor-Recipient		Matched Donor-Recipient		Mismatched Donor-Recipient	
	n	%	n	%	n	hr	n	hr
A1	3	29.4	4	14.2	3	4.6	4	2.4
A2	5	17.9	8	10.1	4	3.4	7	0.6*
A3	7	25.6	2	23.8	6	3.9	0	ND
A24	5	21.5	5	12.6	4	3.0	4	2.1
B7	7	25.6	3	14.4	6	3.9	2	2.2
B8	5	24.0	2	3.8*	5	4.6	2	0.4
Bw44	6	29.3	3	2.4*	6	3.9	3	0.2*
B15	7	25.6	1	21.3	6	3.9	1	1.6
B35	5	30.1	3	17.7	4	4.1	2	0.9
B40	7	25.6	5	12.9	6	3.9	4	2.1
Total	57		36		50		29	

ABBREVIATION: ND = no data.
NOTES: Recipients of matched donor granulocytes had no detectable leukocyte antibodies. Recipients of mismatched donor granulocytes had antibodies detected in one or more of the leukocyte antibody assays.
*p < .01.

dium 111 granulocytes was determined in 36 patients whose sera reacted in one or more of the leukocyte antibody assays and who received normal donor granulocytes containing certain HLA antigens absent in the patient (Table 10–5). When donor and recipient were mismatched for the HLA-A2, B8, or Bw44 antigens, there was a significant reduction in either recovery, t½, or both. Four patients with specific HLA antibodies received granulocytes that contained the corresponding antigens (Table 10–6). In two patients with anti-HLA-A2 and one with anti-HLA-A24, it appears that the recovery of the incompatible cells was reduced and the t½ shortened. Because of the small number of studies, p values were not calculated.

Ninety-three studies also involved indium scans, 45 of which were in patients determined to have localized inflammation at the time of the study. No antibody was detected by any of the five methods in 27 of the 93 studies. GA antibodies were present with other kinds of antibodies in 12 studies (Table 10–7). Six scans were true negatives (no granulocyte localization when inflammation was absent); however, two patients had false negative scans. One had clinically apparent submandibular cellulitis and one had osteomyelitis at a leg amputation stump, but indium granulocytes failed to localize at these sites. A third patient was classified as both false negative and false positive. This 22-year-old female post–renal transplant patient with juvenile-onset diabetes had an intra-abdominal abscess at which indium 111 granulocytes failed to localize (false negative), but pulmonary sequestration of indium 111 granulocytes occurred in the absence of pulmonary inflammation (false positive). Two additional patients with GA antibodies had abnormal pulmonary sequestration of granulocytes and thus were classified as false positives. One was a 72-year-old man with chronic autoimmune neutropenia whose serum reacted in the GA, GC, GIF, and ADLG assays. The intravascular recovery of his granulocytes was reduced to 4.6% and their survival was very short (t½ = 0.2 hours). Severe abnormal bilateral pulmonary uptake of indium 111 granulocytes was apparent throughout the 24 hours following injection. The other patient with a false positive scan was a 9-year-old female post–bone marrow transplantation for acute myelogenous leukemia. Neither of the patients had evidence of pulmonary inflammation and neither was on any drugs likely to cause pulmonary toxicity. All of the patients who had false negative or false

Table 10–6.　　　　　　　　　　**Influence of Specific HLA Antibodies on the Recovery and Half-Life (t½) of Indium 111 Granulocytes**

| | | Patients with Specific HLA Antibodies | | | | | | | | Patients with No Antibodies | | |
| | | Sera Reactivity | | | | | | Recovery (%) | t½ (hr) | | Recovery (%) | t½ (hr) |
Patient	Neutropenic	GA	GC	LC	GIF	ADLG	Antibody			n		
1	Yes	−	−	+	+	+	A2	5.1	0.5	9	10.7	5.4
2	Yes	−	+	+	+	−	A24	2.2	0.2	9	10.7	5.4
3	No	−	−	+	+	−	A2	16.2	1.4	9	30.8	5.6
4	Yes	−	+	+	+	−	A24	26.5	7.4	9	10.7	5.4

Table 10–7. Indium Body Scans in 32 Patients with Detectable Granulocyte Antibodies

Antibody	n	True Neg	True Pos	False Neg	False Pos
GA	4	3	1[b]	None	None
GA + others	12	6	1[b]	2½[c]	2½[c]
GC	12	6	6	None	None
GC + others[a]	12	7	5	None	None
LC	4	2	2	None	None
LC + others[a]	10	None	2	None	None
GIF	1	None	1	None	None
GIF + others[a]	13	11	2	None	None
ADLG	11	5	6	None	None
ADLG + others[a]	9	7	2	None	None

NOTES: Thirty-two patients had antibodies detectable by only one of the five methods. Thirty-four patients were studied with antibodies detected by different combinations of two or more methods. Because the data is grouped to show different combinations of antibodies, the total appears greater.
[a]Excludes GA antibodies.
[b]These two studies were done on the same patient at different times.
[c]Patient classified as both false **positive** and false **negative**

positive scans had serum which reacted in the GA and GIF assays. Many patients whose serum reacted in one or more of the other leukocyte antibody tests had true positive scans and none had false negative or false positive scans. An example of this is shown in Figure 10–3 (see page 124), which is an indium scan of a woman whose serum reacted by granulocytotoxicity against the injected cells, but indium 111 granulocytes localized at the site of a pelvic abscess.

In summary, it appears that immune destruction of granulocytes can best be predicted by the granulocyte agglutination test or possibly more accurately by the combination of GA and GIF tests. The association between lymphocytotoxicity and GIF reactivity, and the observation of reduced recovery and survival when some HLA antigens were mismatched, suggests that LC antibodies and the HLA system are involved in granulocyte destruction. However, routine interpretation of the LC assay is not useful in predicting this. Testing sera by LC against a large number of panel cells might be used to identify highly immunized patients. It is likely that such sera will react by GIF and GA. This may identify patients in whom granulocyte recovery and survival will be reduced.

Figure 10–3.

Indium 111 body scan showing abnormal localization of cells at the site of a pelvic abscess.

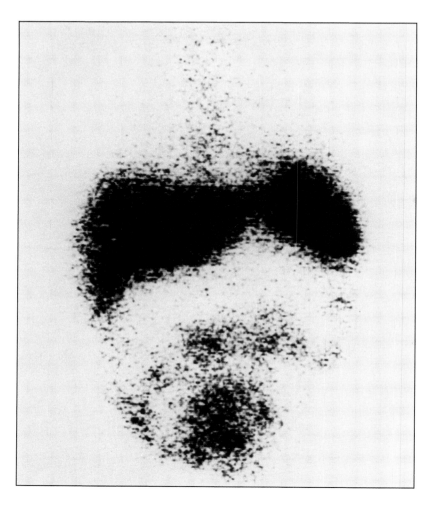

Chapter 11

Case Studies

These case studies are based on patient specimens studied in our laboratory. They have been selected to show approaches for the serologic investigation of various diagnoses related to granulocyte antibodies. In addition, practical applications of some basic methods described in chapter 13 are illustrated.

The *heading* for each case specifies a clinical situation: transfusion reactions (febrile and pulmonary), alloimmune neonatal neutropenia, autoimmune neutropenia (juvenile and adult), and an unidentified antibody in a multiparous donor. These represent the situations most commonly encountered in our laboratory. Following the *purpose*, which identifies the basic techniques or methods exemplified by each case, is a brief *clinical history* and a summary of serologic *results*. The *analysis* explains rationale of testing and interpretation of results. Included in the *comments* are additional observations and guidelines from experience in our laboratory that may be useful to others.

Case 1	*Febrile Transfusion Reaction*

Purpose   Identification of a granulocyte antibody.

Clinical History   A.B., a 76-year-old woman with a history of 15 pregnancies and no previous transfusions, underwent a radical vulvectomy. During surgery, she received one unit of packed red cells without complication. Three days later, a second transfusion of packed red blood cells was begun. After 1 hour the patient experienced chills and headache. A 3°C rise in temperature was noted, and the transfusion was discontinued. Serum samples were referred to our laboratory to determine if granulocyte antibodies were present.

Results

A granulocyte antibody screening was done on the patient's postreaction serum:

Panel Donor	Granulocyte Typing									Serum Reactions			
										GA		GIF	
	NA1	NA2	NB1	NB2	NC1	5a	5b	9a	Mart	1:1	1:4	1:1	1:4
1.	+	+	+	+	+	+	+	+	+	3	3	1	3
2.	+	0	+	0	0	0	+	0	+	3	3	3	3
3.	0	+	0	+	+	+	+	+	+	1	0	0	0
4.	+	+	+	+	+	+	0	+	+	3	1	2	3
5.	0	+	+	+	+	+	+	+	+	1	3	2	3
6.	+	0	+	+	0	0	+	+	+	3	3	3	3
7.	+	+	0	+	+	0	+	+	+	0	0	0	0
8.	+	+	+	0	+	+	+	0	0	2	0	1	3

The limited quantity of prereaction serum permitted testing of only selected cells:

Panel Donor	Granulocyte Typing									Serum Reactions			
										GA		GIF	
	NA1	NA2	NB1	NB2	NC1	5a	5b	9a	Mart	1:1	1:4	1:1	1:4
2.	+	0	+	0	0	0	+	0	+	2	2	2	2
7.	+	+	0	+	+	0	+	+	+	0	0	0	0

The patient's granulocytes were typed in the GA assay:

NA1	NA2	NB1	NB2	NC1	5a	5b	9a	Mart
+	+	0	+	+	0	+	+	+

The postreaction serum was tested for HLA antibodies by lymphocytotoxicity. Results showed that 38 of the 60 cells in the panel were positive, demonstrating multispecificity.

Analysis

The granulocyte antibody screening of the patient's postreaction serum indicated the presence of anti-NB1. The two NB1-negative donors (3 and 7) were the only two nonreactive cells in the GIF assay and were negative or very weakly reactive in GA. All other specificities were excluded at one or both serum dilutions in both assays. The weak reactivity with donor 3 in GA was probably due to the HLA antibodies detected in the LC assay. The presence of anti-NB1 in the prereaction serum was shown using selected cells. The lack of NB1 antigen on the patient's granulocytes confirmed her capability of producing an alloantibody to NB1.

The presence of anti-NB1 in the prereaction serum and the uneventful operative transfusion suggested that the patient had become sensitized during pregnancies, but her antibody level had diminished with time. The initial transfusion probably produced a rapid rise in antibody titer due to anamnestic response, which caused the febrile reaction to the second transfusion.

Comments

1. The prozone phenomenon has been observed in the GA assay. Therefore, sera are tested both undiluted and at a dilution. Elimination of either of these can cause confusion in antibody identification. While true prozoning does not occur in a direct binding assay like GIF, a similar effect has been noted, and the two serum dilutions are also used for antibody screening in GIF.

2. As febrile reactions are most often attributed to antibodies in the recipient[7,237] and such an antibody was detected, the donors' sera were not tested in this case. The high frequency of the NB1 antigen (97%) makes the probability of one or both donors being NB1-positive quite likely.

3. As seen with this case, testing of the patient's prereaction and postreaction serum may aid in determining the etiology of the reaction. However, prereaction serum is often depleted by the red blood cell serologic transfusion reaction testing.

4. Although NB1 and NB2 are reported to be alleles,[61] no dosage effect has been observed with antibodies to NB1 in GA or GIF.

5. Sera from febrile transfusion reactions are not routinely screened for granulocyte antibodies at our institution. In a study of 55 sera from such reactions, no correlation was found between the presence of granulocyte agglutinins and the rise in temperature. The predictive values of other assays for febrile reactions have not been investigated.

Case 2 | **Pulmonary Transfusion Reaction**

Purpose

Differentiation of granulocyte and HLA antibodies using platelet absorption.

F.D., a previously untransfused, 73-year-old man, underwent surgery for the elective repair of an aortic abdominal aneurysm. Intraoperatively he received nine units of whole blood and two units of fresh frozen plasma without complication. Within 2 hours of surgery, the patient experienced acute pulmonary distress and leukopenia (WBC = 0.4×10^9 per liter). Although severe, the symptoms resolved with respiratory support and intense steroid therapy.[23]

Results

Sera from nine of the 11 donors, as well as postreaction serum from the patient, were obtained and tested for granulocyte and HLA (LC) antibodies. (Prereaction serum from the recipient was unavailable.) Eight of nine donors' sera and that of the patient showed no reactivity in GA or GIF when tested with an eight-cell panel, or in LC with 28 cells. Serum from the last whole-blood donor (V.P.) reacted in GA and GIF, as well as demonstrating anti-Bw44 in the LC assay. Because an HLA antibody was present, V.P.'s serum was absorbed with platelets and found to be negative in LC postabsorption.

Granulocyte testing showed the following reactivity:

Panel Donor	Granulocyte Typing									V.P.'s Serum Reactions							
										GA				GIF			
										Unabsorbed		Plt-absorbed		Unabsorbed		Plt-absorbed	
	NA1	NA2	NB1	NB2	NC1	5a	5b	9a	Mart	1:1	1:4	1:1	1:4	1:1	1:4	1:1	1:4
1.	0	+	+	0	+	+	0	0	+	4	3	4	3	4	4	4	4
2.	+	+	+	+	+	0	+	+	+	4	4	4	3	4	3	4	3
3.	+	0	+	+	0	+	+	+	+	3	1	0	0	0	2	0	0
4.	0	+	0	+	+	+	+	+	+	4	3	4	3	4	4	4	4
5.	+	0	+	0	0	+	+	0	+	0	0	0	0	0	0	0	0
6.	+	0	+	0	0	0	+	0	+	0	0	0	0	0	0	0	0
7.	+	+	+	+	+	+	+	+	0	4	3	3	3	4	4	4	3
8.	+	+	0	+	+	0	+	+	+	3	2	3	2	4	3	4	3

The patient's cells were typed in the GA assay and tested with V.P.'s serum:

	Granulocyte Typing									HLA	Typing
Cells:	NA1	NA2	NB1	NB2	NC1	5a	5b	9a	Mart	A	B
F.D.	+	+	+	0	+	+	+	0	+	2,28	13,w51

	Serum: V.P. (1:1, 1:4)		
Cells:	GA	GIF	LC
F.D.	4	4	0

Testing of the patient's cells with the sera of the other eight donors was nonreactive in GA, GIF, and LC.

Analysis	Because some cases of severe pulmonary transfusion reaction have been attributed to passively transfused granulocyte or HLA antibodies,[23,67,239,242] attempts were made to obtain serum from all donors for screening for both granulocyte and HLA antibodies. The granulocyte antibody detected in the unabsorbed serum of donor V.P. was suggestive of anti-NA2, as two of three NA2-negative panel cells were nonreactive. Following platelet absorption to remove the HLA anti-Bw44, the reactivity with the third NA2-negative donor was absent, confirming the antibody as anti-NA2. Panel donor 3 was positive for Bw44. Minor crossmatches, consisting of testing patients' cells and donors' sera, provided additional evidence implicating the anti-NA2 in the reaction. The cells of F.D. were NA2-positive, lacked Bw44, and reacted with V.P.'s serum in GA and GIF but not with LC.

Comments

1. It may not be feasible in some cases to obtain serum specimens from donors. CPD-A1 plasma from segments has been used in our laboratory for granulocyte screening if hemolysis is minimal. However, as the small quantity of plasma obtained from segments precludes recalcification, the complement-dependent LC assay cannot be performed, nor can platelet absorption be attempted. Therefore, the more informative results obtained from serum specimens often make the effort to collect them worthwhile.

2. Due to the high degree of polymorphism in the HLA system, LC typing and/or crossmatching with patients' cells is necessary to support any causal relationship of HLA antibodies to transfusion reactions. HLA antibodies detected in donor sera may not be directed to antigens on patients' cells. Although most granulocyte antigens occur with relatively high frequencies, typing the recipient's granulocytes is still desirable.

3. While obtaining sufficient cells for typing and crossmatching from a nonneutropenic patient is not difficult, the timing and collection conditions are critical. Therefore, early communication and coordination with the laboratory performing testing is essential.

4. Testing in cases of pulmonary transfusion reactions often produces less informative results than described in this case. The acute posttransfusion leukopenia in this patient appeared to be significant. When documented, such leukopenia may indicate cases particularly suitable for granulocyte serologic study.

Alloimmune Neonatal Neutropenia (ANN)

Purpose	Utilization of a family study in diagnosis of neutropenia.

Clinical History	E.W. was admitted to the hospital 2 weeks after birth for evaluation of unexplained buttock pustules and circumcision infection. Upon admission, his white blood cell count was 10.9×10^9 per liter, with 9% neutrophils and no other hematologic abnormalities. Two days later, he developed profound neutropenia with 0% circulating neutrophils. The infections resolved with antibiotic therapy, and he was maintained on prophylactic antibiotics until his absolute neutrophil count returned to normal levels at age 2 months.

Results	Serum from both the infant and his mother were tested for antibodies:

Panel Donor	Granulocyte Typing									Serum Reactions							
										Infant				Mother			
										GA		GIF		GA		GIF	
	NA1	NA2	NB1	NB2	NC1	5a	5b	9a	Mart	1:1	1:4	1:1	1:4	1:1	1:4	1:1	1:4
1.	+	0	+	+	0	0	+	+	+	1	0	2	0	4	3	4	4
2.	0	+	0	+	+	+	+	+	+	0	0	0	0	0	0	0	0
3.	+	+	+	+	+	+	+	+	+	0	0	1	0	3	2	4	4
4.	+	0	+	0	0	0	+	0	+	2	0	2	1	3	3	4	4
5.	0	+	+	0	+	0	+	0	+	0	0	0	0	0	0	0	0
6.	+	+	+	+	+	+	+	+	0	1	0	2	0	3	2	4	4
7.	+	+	0	+	+	0	+	+	+	0	0	0	0	3	2	4	3
8.	0	+	+	+	+	+	0	+	+	0	0	0	0	0	0	0	0

Lymphocytotoxic antibodies were not detected in serum from the mother or infant.

The granulocytes of the parents were typed and tested with serum from the mother and infant:

Cells	Granulocyte Typing									Serum (1:1)			
										Infant		Mother	
	NA1	NA2	NB1	NB2	NC1	5a	5b	9a	Mart	GA	GIF	GA	GIF
Mother	0	+	+	+	+	0	+	+	+	0	0	0	0
Father	+	0	+	+	0	+	+	+	+	2	2	4	4

ANN should be considered in an infant less than 4 to 6 months of age with unexplained neutropenia and without documentation of a previous normal absolute neutrophil count. Since the quantity of available serum from an infant is generally limited, and antibody levels may be low due to adsorption onto the infant's granulocytes, testing of maternal serum is informative. This mother's serum demonstrated strong anti-NA1 activity in both assays. Though weaker, reactivity in the infant's serum was also suggestive of anti-NA1. These results were consistent with ANN. Because this was their first child, the parents were concerned about the possibility of ANN occurring in future pregnancies. Typing of the parents' granulocytes indicated all offspring would be heterozygous NA1-positive. Crossmatching of maternal and infant sera with parents' granulocytes provided further evidence for the potential for maternal sensitization during pregnancy, and demonstrated no maternal autoantibodies.

Comments

1. Maternal antibodies in cases of ANN often provide an excellent source of reagent antisera. Such healthy women should be encouraged to contribute plasma.

2. Many maternal sera contain HLA antibodies. When possible, such sera should be absorbed with random pooled platelets or with paternal cells obtained from the mononuclear layer of the double-density gradient before testing with the father's granulocytes.

3. When the maternal serum is nonreactive with a panel of normal donors, crossmatching with paternal granulocytes is important to exclude an antibody to a low-incidence antigen.

4. Obtaining adequate granulocytes for typing and crossmatching from a neutropenic infant is usually not feasible and not required for diagnosis of ANN.

Case 4   Juvenile Autoimmune Neutropenia (AIN)

Purpose

Confirmation of granulocyte antibody identity using granulocyte absorption.

Clinical History

L.J., a 13-month-old female, had been well until she presented with fever, otitis media, and an erythematous skin nodule on the cheek, thought to be an insect bite. Persistence of the nodule led to CBC testing, showing a WBC = 5.1×10^9 per liter, with 2% neutrophils, and diagnosis of a mandibular abscess. The infections resolved with antibiotic therapy, but neutropenia has persisted for 10 months.

Initial testing of the patient's serum showed the following results:

Panel Donor	Granulocyte Typing NA1	NA2	NB1	NB2	NC1	5a	5b	9a	Mart	Serum Reactions GA 1:1	1:4	GIF 1:1	1:4
1.	+	0	+	+	0	0	+	+	+	3	2	2	3
2.	0	+	+	+	+	0	+	+	+	3	0	2	2
3.	0	+	+	0	+	0	+	0	+	3	1	3	3
4.	+	+	0	0	+	+	+	0	+	3	2	3	3
5.	+	0	+	+	0	0	+	+	+	3	2	3	3
6.	+	+	+	+	+	+	+	+	0	3	3	3	3
7.	+	+	+	0	+	+	0	+	+	3	3	2	3
8.	0	+	0	+	+	0	+	+	+	3	1	3	3

Lymphocytotoxicity testing was negative.

The patient's serum was absorbed with normal NA1-positive and NA1-negative granulocytes and retested with selected cells:

Panel Donor	Granulocyte Typing NA1	NA2	NB1	NB2	NC1	5a	5b	9a	Mart	Serum Reactions GA (Serum diluted 1:4) Unabsorbed	*NA1-pos	*NA1 neg	GIF (Serum diluted 1:4) Unabsorbed	*NA1-pos	*NA1-neg
9.	+	+	0	+	+	0	+	+	+	3	0	3	3	3	3
10.	0	+	+	+	+	0	+	+	+	1	0	0	3	3	3

* Absorbing cell type.

The antibody was titrated with NA1-positive and NA1-negative panel cells:

Panel Cell	Titer GA	GIF
NA1-positive	64	256
NA1-negative	8	128

Testing of the patient's serum and normal NA1-positive granulocytes in GIF with monospecific conjugates showed the following results:

FITC- Conjugated Antihuman Globulin	Reaction
IgG	3
IgM	1
IgA	0

Sufficient granulocytes could not be obtained from the patient's blood for direct testing and typing.

Analysis

Initial testing of the patient's serum showed weaker reactions with NA1-negative donors at a 1:4 dilution in the GA assay. GIF results suggested no specificity. As LC antibodies were not detected and the volume of serum was limited, granulocyte rather than platelet absorption was performed. In GA, the reactivity with an NA1-positive cell (donor 9) was completely removed by absorption with cells expressing NA1 and unaffected by absorption with cells lacking that antigen. This is consistent with anti-NA1 in the patient's serum. Weaker reactivity against NA1-negative cells was removed by absorption with cells of either type, indicative of a high-frequency granulocyte antibody of undetermined specificity. Absorptions showed no effect on reactions in GIF.

Titrations demonstrated further evidence of the presence of anti-NA1. The GA titer was significantly higher with NA1-positive cells, while the GIF titer was not. In addition, the titers provided reference points for later testing of the patient's antibody levels.

Monospecific GIF testing indicated the antibody was predominantly IgG with a lesser IgM component. This was consistent with a relatively early phase of AIN, supported by unresolved neutropenia during the 10 months the patient has been followed.

Comments

1. Demonstration of antibody specificity in only one assay is not uncommon in AIN and emphasizes the value of testing with more than one type of assay.

2. While granulocyte absorption can be informative, caution in interpretation of results must be exercised. Some autoantibodies that have an apparent specificity can be absorbed by antigen-negative cells, similar to the phenomenon sometimes seen in red blood cell serology with red blood cell autoantibodies (see the section on autoantibodies v alloantibodies in chapter 5).

3. Compared to alloantibodies, specificities of autoantibodies are generally less distinct and may become more obscure during the course of the disease.

Adult Autoimmune Neutropenia (AIN)

Purpose   Interpretation of direct granulocyte immunofluorescence.

Clinical History   P.M., a 58-year-old woman, was evaluated for neutropenia of 2 years' duration. During this period, her absolute neutrophil count was 0.8 to 1.2 $\times$ 10^9 per liter, with her primary complaint being numerous upper respiratory infections. She had a history of four pregnancies, and had been transfused following a hysterectomy 5 years previously. The day of serologic testing, her white count was 5.4 $\times$ 10^9 per liter, with 15% neutrophils.

Results   The patient's serum was screened for granulocyte antibodies:

Panel Donor	Granulocyte Typing									Serum Reactions			
										GA		GIF	
	NA1	NA2	NB1	NB2	NC1	5a	5b	9a	Mart	1:1	1:4	1:1	1:4
1.	+	0	+	+	0	+	+	+	+	1	0	0	0
2.	+	+	+	0	+	0	+	0	+	2	1	3	2
3.	0	+	+	+	+	0	+	+	+	2	2	3	3
4.	+	+	0	+	+	+	+	+	+	2	2	3	2
5.	+	0	+	0	0	0	+	0	+	0	0	0	0
6.	0	+	+	+	+	+	0	+	+	2	2	3	3
7.	0	+	0	+	+	0	+	+	+	2	2	3	3
8.	+	0	+	+	0	0	+	+	+	1	0	0	0

The antibody was titrated with cells of donor 4 showing titers of 16 (GA) and 256 (GIF). Lymphocytotoxic testing was negative.

The patient's whole blood was obtained for direct granulocyte testing in GIF, using FITC-conjugated antihuman total immunoglobulin, IgG, IgM, and IgA:

Serum	Patient's Granulocytes				Normal Control Granulocytes			
	Total Ig	IgG	IgM	IgA	Total Ig	IgG	IgM	IgA
Positive control	4	4	2	2	4	4	2	2
Negative control	1	2	0	0	0	0	0	0
Autologous	1	2	0	0	0	0	0	0
None (direct)	2	2	0	0	0	0	0	0

The patient's granulocytes were also typed in GA:

NA1	NA2	NB1	NB2	NC1	5a	5b	9a	Mart	Auto Control
+	+	+	0	+	0	+	0	+	0

Analysis

Testing of the patient's serum indicated the presence of anti-NA2. Although some weak nonspecific reactivity was seen with undiluted serum with donors 1 and 8 in GA, results at 1:4 and in GIF clearly define the specificity. Since the patient had a history of both pregnancy and transfusion, it was necessary to test the patient's granulocytes to determine whether the anti-NA2 was an alloantibody or autoantibody. Typing of the granulocytes indicated it was autoimmune.

Direct testing further substantiated the presence of an autoantibody. In examining normal donor granulocytes, reactivity with positive control sera and no reactions with negative or auto controls or direct testing indicate appropriate dilutions of each of the conjugates. Reactivity of the patient's cells in the direct tests with total Ig and IgG conjugates indicates the presence of IgG antibody bound in vivo to her granulocytes. The in vivo–bound antibody is also detected in the negative control test.

Comments

1. While it cannot be used for direct testing and may be less sensitive for autologous testing, the GA assay is also less likely to reflect in vivo–bound antibody in typing reactions than GIF. Therefore, even patients with positive direct tests may often be validly typed in GA.

2. GIF reactivity of the patient's serum and cells *in vitro* may be stronger than in the direct test. As this can be helpful in interpretation of weakly positive direct tests, autologous testing should be included whenever possible.

3. The appropriate dilution for each conjugate must be determined by checkerboard titration (see procedure 2.4) before testing with patient cells. Testing normal control granulocytes in parallel with those of the patient verifies the accuracy of the dilution.

4. IgG conjugates often show slightly stronger reactivity than total Ig. However, we have found several granulocyte antibodies consisting of IgM only. Therefore, we continue to use total Ig conjugates for antibody screening.

Unidentified Granulocyte Antibody in the Serum of a Multiparous Woman

Purpose   Characterization of a new granulocyte specificity.

Clinical History   Two days following the birth of her fourth child, the serum of B.M. was tested for granulocyte antibodies in conjunction with an established postpartum screening program to procure HLA and granulocyte serologic reagents. Her medical history was unremarkable, including no hematologic abnormalities. Although white counts and differentials were not done at birth, none of her children experienced any notable illnesses during infancy.

Results   Initial testing of this woman's serum showed strong reactivity with all donors in GA and GIF. Further studies were performed (as discussed in chapter 8) to determine if this antibody defined a previously unidentified granulocyte antigen.

Antibody Screening

Assay	No. Cells Reacting	No. Cells Tested
GA	24	24
GIF	24	24
Red blood cell antiglobulin test	0	10
Lymphocytotoxicity:		
T-lymphocyte	0	60
B-lymphocyte	0	20
Platelet immunofluorescence	0	4

Population Study   The serum was screened with 343 random donors in the GA assay, and reacted with 340.

Antigen frequency = .991
Gene frequency = .906

Two-by-two contingency tables were constructed for each known granulocyte antigen using results obtained by testing the serum with 100 typed random donors in the following way:

		Unknown Antigen	
		Positive	Negative
Known Antigen	Positive	A	B
	Negative	C	D

(A + B + C + D = 100)

Results were statistically evaluated using Fisher's exact test and correlation coefficients:

	Fisher's P	Correlation Coefficient r
NA1	.34	.05
NA2	.45	.18
NB1	.41	.06
NB2	.24	.29
NC1	1.00	—
ND1	1.00	—
5a	.34	.07
5b	.63	.13
9a	.25	.29

Family members were typed for granulocyte, red blood cell, and HLA antigens. Representative results are illustrated in the following pedigree:

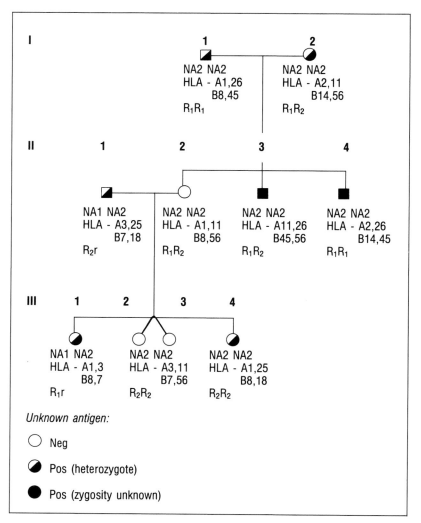

The granulocytes of B.M. (II.2) were typed:

NA1	NA2	NB1	NB2	NC1	ND1	NE1	5a	5b	9a	Auto
0	+	+	+	+	+	0	0	+	+	0

Absorption Studies

Cell line distribution

The serum was absorbed with various purified cell suspensions obtained from donors reactive with the serum and retested:

Cells Used for Absorption	Post-Absorption GA Results with Reactive Donor
Platelets	+
Erythrocytes	+
Monocytes	0
T-lymphocytes	0
B-lymphocytes	+
Granulocytes	0

Following absorption with similar preparations from a non-reactive donor, no change in reactivity was seen.

Determination of monospecificity of the antibody

The serum was absorbed with granulocytes from ten donors and retested with the same donors in GA:

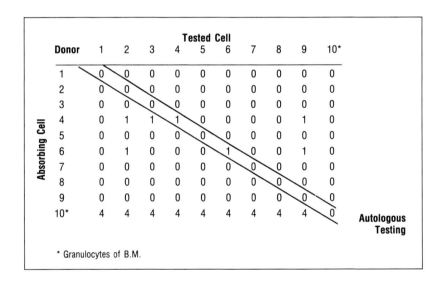

Absorbing Cell \ Donor	Tested Cell 1	2	3	4	5	6	7	8	9	10*
1	0	0	0	0	0	0	0	0	0	0
2	0	0	0	0	0	0	0	0	0	0
3	0	0	0	0	0	0	0	0	0	0
4	0	1	1	1	0	0	0	0	1	0
5	0	0	0	0	0	0	0	0	0	0
6	0	1	0	0	0	1	0	0	1	0
7	0	0	0	0	0	0	0	0	0	0
8	0	0	0	0	0	0	0	0	0	0
9	0	0	0	0	0	0	0	0	0	0
10*	4	4	4	4	4	4	4	4	4	0

Autologous Testing

* Granulocytes of B.M.

Analysis The serum was tested in assays with granulocytes, lymphocytes, erythrocytes, and platelets to determine if other contaminating antibodies were present, or if the unknown antibody reacted directly with other cell lines. The antibody appeared to define a high-frequency antigen on granulocytes. As reactivity in GA and GIF was parallel, most additional studies were done with GA, which requires less serum and is easier to perform with large numbers of donors. However, family studies and testing of antigen-negative donors were done with both assays.

The serum was tested with a large group of random donors to determine the frequency of the antigen in the population. The gene frequency was then calculated, assuming a biallelic system. This gene frequency (.906) was then compared with those of known antigens and their alleles or hypothetical alleles. For example, the gene frequency excluded identity of the unknown antigen with NA1 (.32), but the possibility remained of allelism with NE1 (.12).

The possibility of identity or allelism with known granulocyte antigens was further evaluated statistically using two-by-two contingency tables. Values considered to be statistically significant were P less than .05 and r greater than .30. No significant associations to known antigens were detected in this way.

Reactions with typed donors were further examined for allelism. In a biallelic system, one or both alleles will be expressed in any individual. Two donors were found who lacked both the unknown antigen and NE1. Although the gene frequencies suggested allelism, this excluded that possibility.

The pedigree was examined to evaluate inheritance of the unknown antigen. The gene controlling the production of the antigen cannot be Y-linked because females express the antigen, nor can it be X-linked because the father of the propositus I. 1. passes an x chromosome to the propositus II. 2. without the gene for the unknown antigen. The pattern observed is consistent with autosomal dominant inheritance. Recombination observed for this gene and NA, Rh, and HLA indicate that it is probably not closely linked to any of these loci.

Typing of the granulocytes of the antibody producer excluded alloantibody production to any antigens expressed on her cells. No evidence was found of autoantibodies.

Removal of the antibody following absorptions with monocytes, T-lymphocytes, and granulocytes indicates the expression of the unknown antigen on these cells. Platelets, erythrocytes, and B-lymphocytes did not appear to express the unknown antigen. While other tissues have been used for absorption studies, these cells were selected for their availability from peripheral blood.

Particularly with a high-frequency antibody, the possibility exists that it consists of two or more antibodies. If this were the case, reactivity would have been absorbed to varying degrees by the granulocytes of the nine reactive donors. However, the antibody was uniformly absorbed by all cells, with the exception of the remaining weak reactivity after absorption with cells of donors 4 and 6. This was due to incomplete absorption, indicated by similar reactions in autologous postabsorption testing. Uniform absorption by all nine reactive granulocytes indicates a monospecific, rather than multispecific, antibody.

These studies indicated the antibody in B.M.'s serum did recognize a previously undefined antigen expressed on granulocytes. It was tentatively named Mart, and additional studies were reported.[210]

Comments

1. Granulocyte reactivity in many sera shows no correlation with previously defined antigens. However, some characteristics make extensive investigation, as described here, more feasible:

    a. Strong reactivity at a titer ≥ 16.

    b. Availability of sufficient quantities of serum for investigation and potential future distribution for reagent use.

    c. Antigen frequency between .200 and .800.

    d. Absence of HLA antibodies.

2. Correlation with clinical conditions and/or granulocyte function may be made by obtaining careful medical histories from antibody producers and their families.

Part II

Laboratory Practice

Chapter 12

Implementation of Granulocyte Serology Testing

Resources Required

Laboratory Space

The minimum laboratory space required to accommodate one technologist and the equipment necessary for granulocyte antibody testing is between 100 and 200 square feet. It may be feasible to share this space with another activity compatible in terms of equipment and general activities, such as platelet antibody or histocompatibility testing.

Some of the mechanical resources that must be available include sufficient electrical outlets for the equipment, running water, and hand-washing facilities. Space must be allocated for a desk, supply storage, necessary equipment, and laboratory bench area. The bench space required for most of the actual performance of granulocyte antibody testing techniques is approximately 4 to 6 running feet for each technologist. If granulocyte immunofluorescence is to be used, access to a dark room or curtained area is required for using the fluorescence microscope. There should also be sufficient uncontaminated space available to draw blood from panel donors in a private and comfortable atmosphere.

Because storage of files and records can consume substantial space, computerization of files is recommended. However, because of legal considerations, there must be provisions made for storage, off-site or on-site, of the original paper documents. These documents include test requests, patient data forms, panels, and reports from specimen testing in addition to records of donors and antisera used in testing.

Equipment

The equipment required for granulocyte antibody testing is not extensive. However, since some of it is relatively expensive, great care should be taken in its selection, and the possibility of sharing existing equipment should be thoroughly explored. Below is a list of the major items of equipment that will be required for the installation of granulocyte antibody testing using granulocyte agglutination and immunofluorescence assays. (Smaller items of equipment such as microliter pipets and syringes are not included.)

Equipment Required	Approximate Cost ($)
Fluorescence microscope with phase contrast	20,000
Microcentrifuge	1,200
Refrigerated laboratory centrifuge	6,600
Tube rotator	150
Vortex mixer	200
pH Meter	750
Analytical balance	600
Refrigerator	700
Laboratory freezer	4,000
Water bath	700
Incubators (2)	2,000
Cell counter	3,000
Total cost	**39,900**

Personnel

Granulocyte antibody testing is labor-intensive and exacting, in performance of actual testing procedures and in preparatory and supportive activities.

The nature of granulocyte antibody testing is such that it requires technologists with some prior experience in immunohematological assays and technical problem solving. Careful attention to detail is critical for accurate performance of assays and interpretation of results.

Services of a physician familiar with the medical aspects of the diagnosis, treatment of patients with immune neutropenias, and management of patients suffering from transfusion reactions is a great asset. The physician should (1) monitor the reports issued by the laboratory, (2) be available for consultation with clinicians requesting laboratory services or advice regarding patient management, (3) provide scientific leadership regarding technical problems and development, and (4) monitor the overall activity of the laboratory.

We currently test approximately 700 specimens each year (both clinical and research) with a standard protocol (see Testing Protocol). Two full time technologists are required to perform these tests and the related activities to support this testing.

Although some items vary from week-to-week, the average allocation of the technologists' time is itemized below:

Activity	Hrs/Week Per Tech	Percentage of Time
Testing	15.5	41.3
Testing Preparation	10.5	28.0
Reporting/Billing	2.8	7.5
Data Evaluation	1.9	5.1
Manuscripts/Correspondence	1.6	4.2
Methods Development	1.5	4.0
Reagent Preparation	1.0	2.7
Special Studies	.8	2.1
Training	.9	2.4
Presentations	1.0	2.7
Total	**37.5**	**100.0**

As illustrated above, 41.3% of the total technologist time is spent on performance testing. 30.7% is required for test and reagent preparation. Also, 7.5% of their time is required for reporting and billing and 4.0% is needed for methods development and solving problems that arise with the assays. Therefore, a total of 83.5% of technologist time is spent on testing samples or on other sample-related activities.

This leaves 16.5% of technologist time available for other activities. In our laboratory, this is spent on a variety of developmental projects; training of residents, fellows and technologists; continuing education presentations; preparation of manuscripts; and data evaluation activities.

These figures can be used as guidelines for the approximate amount of technologist time required for granulocyte antibody testing. Adjustments to these figures are required for the number of specimens tested, experience of technologists, and assays performed. Substantial reduction in the number of specimens tested would decrease the time required. However, certain aspects of testing, such as granulocyte isolation and incubations, require a fixed amount of time. The two technologists represented in this time study were experienced in performing these assays. A technologist who is just beginning to learn these assays will, of course, require more time to accomplish the same amount of testing. These figures also are based on the testing scheme that we use in our laboratory, which includes testing each sample concurrently by granulocyte agglutination and granulocyte immunofluorescence with both un-absorbed and platelet-absorbed serum (if necessary).

Implementation of Granulocyte Antibody Testing

Testing Protocol

The plethora of available methods for the detection of granulocyte antibodies requires that careful selection be made for the establishment of a serology program. The feasibility of setting up an in-house granulocyte laboratory versus using the services of a reference laboratory will, to some extent, depend on the volume of work, the available staff, and access to a population of individuals for use as dependable panel donors. For our serology program, we have chosen the granulocyte agglutination (GA) and granulocyte immunofluorescence (GIF) assays as our two basic methods for antigen typing and antibody detection. The GA method (1) has historically been the reference method for the identification of granulocyte antigens involved in alloimmune and autoimmune neutropenias; (2) requires very small volumes (3μl) of serum for antigen typing, which makes it feasible to type large numbers of individuals with limited quantities of typing reagents; and (3) detects all of the currently known N series of granulocyte antigens plus 9a. The GIF technique (1) has been shown to be more sensitive, (2) permits detection of antibody immunoglobulin class, and (3) can be used for direct antibody testing. The general characteristics of each method are compared in Table 12–1.

Granulocyte agglutinins are often, but not always, detectable in the GIF test.[81] Conversely, there are antibodies which are detected by GIF but are nonreactive by GA.[61] We believe this phenomenon to be similar to the different reaction pattern observed with different red blood cell antibody detection techniques. Therefore, a thorough examination of specimens requires the use of both techniques.[20,60]

The antibody testing protocol we employ in our laboratory was developed to maximize efficient use of resources (panel donors and technical personnel) while minimizing time between receipt of specimen and final reporting of results (Figure 12–1). Serum samples are routinely tested in the GA and GIF assays against granulocytes from eight normal donors, whose granulocytes are typed for at least the following granulocyte antigens: NA1, NA2, NB1, NB2, NC1, 5a, 5b, 9a, and Mart. Testing with additional panel cells is done as necessary to identify or exclude antibodies to these antigens.

Because HLA antibodies also react in both of these assays, serum reactive in either GA or GIF is tested for HLA antibodies by LC. The serum is screened against a panel of 24 selected lymphocyte populations that are positive for the major HLA-A, HLA-B, and HLA-C antigens. If HLA antibodies are detected, the serum is ab-

Table 12–1. **Characteristics Associated with Granulocyte Agglutination (GA) and Granulocyte Immunofluorescence (GIF) Assays**

Test	Reagent volume per test Serum (μL)	Cells (×10³)	Immunoglobulin Class Determination	Time Required* (hr) Cell Prep	Assay	Total	Interpretation of Results	Advantages	Disadvantages
GA	3	5	No	1.2	4.3	5.5	Microscopic observation of clumping	Simple Small serum requirement Reproducible Requires less capital investment and equipment	Not as sensitive Not all antibodies detectable by GA Cannot be used for direct antibody testing
GIF	20	200	Yes	1.3	2.3	3.6	Qualitative evaluation of cellular fluorescence by microscopy	Sensitive Results can be quantitated Applicable for indirect and direct antibody body testing Quantitative measurement of cellular fluorescence by cytofluorometry	Interpretation of results is more subjective; requires more operator experience Immune complexes and nonspecific Ig binding can interfere with test interpretation Requires fluorescence microscope Not all antibodies detected by GIF

*As determined for 50 tests with one cell preparation.

sorbed with washed, pooled platelets to remove this activity. In situations involving very weakly reactive GA or GIF antibodies or limited amounts of serum, platelet absorption may not be feasible. In this situation, lymphocytes from the granulocyte donors who were positive with the patient specimen can be tested with the same serum using the LC assay to evaluate the contribution of possible HLA activity to the positive granulocyte reaction.

Following platelet absorption, serum is retested in GA and/or GIF. Reactivity in these assays after complete HLA absorptions suggests the presence of granulocyte-specific antibodies. To conserve time and prevent substantial delays in reporting, sera reactive in GA and/or GIF may be absorbed with platelets prior to initial LC testing, as depicted in Figure 12–1. Absorbed and unabsorbed sera are then tested in parallel in the GA, GIF, and LC assays concurrently. The interpretation and distinction of antibody reactivity in the GA and GIF assay is shown in Table 12–2. Specimens

Figure 12–1.

Granulocyte antibody detection testing protocol.

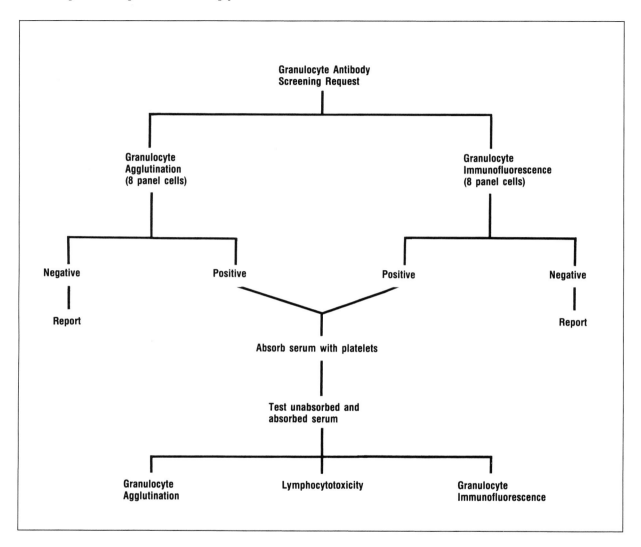

are tested in the GC and ADLG assays in cases suggestive of cytotoxic or cellular immune mechanisms. These procedures are available through our research laboratory but are not routinely utilized for antibody testing.

Antibody prozone is frequently observed in granulocyte antibody testing and especially in the GA assay. Therefore, we screen all of our specimens undiluted and at a 1:5 dilution. In the GA assay, prolonged incubation can result in cell lysis. Cells in wells containing undiluted serum are more prone to cell damage, and thus it is important to read the results after 4 or 5 hours of incubation.

Table 12-2.

**Granulocyte Antibody Reactions After Evaluation by
Lymphocytotoxicity (LC)**

Serum	Granulocyte Antibody Reaction	LC	Interpretation
Unabsorbed	+	+	None
Absorbed	0	0	HLA Antibody
Unabsorbed	+	+	HLA Antibody
Absorbed	+	0	+ Granulocyte-specific antibody
Unabsorbed	+	0	Granulocyte-specific antibody
Absorbed	+	0	None

Although it has been indicated that ABO antigens do not interfere with either GA or GIF testing,[56,81] our panel donors are predominantly group O to eliminate any possibility of interfering isohemagglutinin activity.

When indicated, patient granulocytes are typed by GA for the same antigens as previously mentioned for the panel donors. Qualitative determination of in vivo cell-associated immunoglobulin on patients' granulocytes can be accomplished using conjugated antibodies to total immunoglobulins, IgG, IgM, and IgA in the GIF assay.

Descriptions of the granulocyte isolation, GA, GIF, and platelet-absorption techniques are provided in chapter 13.

Specimen Requirements

For granulocyte antibody testing, 5 to 10 mL of serum is usually sufficient. Limited testing may be done on as little as 1 mL of serum. Blood should be drawn into tubes without any separation medium. Serum should be separated from red blood cells as soon as possible and stored at $-80°C$ until tested. After thawing, it may be necessary to clarify the serum with high-speed centrifugation to remove any debris present prior to testing.

Granulocyte typing and direct antibody testing must be performed within 24 hours of venipuncture. Disodium edetate (Na_2 EDTA) is the anticoagulant of choice. Alternatively, the following anticoagulant mixture may be used when available to provide better maintenance of granulocyte viability during shipment or for delayed testing:

9.0 mL	Whole blood
1.0 mL	CPD or CPD-A1
0.1 mL	10% Na_2 EDTA

It is critical that blood samples for granulocyte isolation be maintained at room temperature (20° to 24°C) until tested. When patient granulocytes are needed for testing, it must be remembered that granulocytes obtained from an individual in an abnormal condition may not behave as normal granulocytes on density separation gradients. The volume of blood required to provide sufficient granulocytes depends upon absolute neutrophil count (Table 2–5). The various specimens needed for investigations involving suspected cases of alloimmune neonatal neutropenia, autoimmune neutropenia, febrile and pulmonary transfusion reactions, and drug-associated agranulocytosis are described in Table 12–3.

The establishment of a granulocyte panel and the associated techniques needed for accurate detection of granulocyte antibodies requires a substantial commitment of personnel and resources. The cost-effectiveness of setting up such a program must be weighed against using the facilities of reference laboratories. Both have their own distinct advantages, so the decision tends to focus on the amount of work generated, the availability of needed equipment, and the access to laboratories for assistance in the detection of

Table 12–3. **Specimen Requirements for Granulocyte Antibody Detection Testing**

Condition	Specimen Needed		Type of Specimen Needed	
		Serum	EDTA Anticoagulated Blood[a]	Heparin Anticoagulated Blood[b]
Autoimmune neutropenia	Acute	X[c]	X if ANC > 1000	NA
	Convalescent	X	X	NA
Alloimmune neonatal neutropenia	Infant	X	NA	NA
	Mother	X	X	X
	Father	X	X	X
Transfusion Reaction	Patient: prereaction	X	NA	NA
	1-week postreaction	X	X	X
	Donor	X	X	NA
Drug-associated neutropenia	Acute	X[d]	NA	NA
	Convalescent	X	X	NA

ABBREVIATIONS: ANC = absolute neutrophil count; NA = not applicable.
[a]For isolation of granulocytes (granulocyte typing, crossmatching or direct antibody testing).
[b]For isolation of lymphocytes (lymphocytes HLA typing or crossmatching).
[c]Preferably drawn before initiation of steroid therapy.
[d]Drawn within two days of drug discontinuation.

contaminating HLA antibodies or immune complexes. Laboratories with limited resources may choose to screen patient sera for granulocyte antibodies while using a reference laboratory for antibody identification or special studies.

Typing Reagents

Procurement

As it is difficult to obtain enough reagent-quality antisera independently, it is important to establish serum exchange programs with other laboratories doing granulocyte antibody testing. These reagents are absolutely necessary for typing granulocytes to be used as screening cells, or on antibody identification panels, or for use as known antibodies in evaluating new granulocyte antibody detection tests.

We have found that random screening of large populations of potentially immunized people is not a cost-effective means of obtaining these reagents.[164] In testing the sera from 2,313 multiparous female donors, we found lymphocytotoxins in the sera of 397 (14.2%) and granulocyte agglutinins in the sera of 291 (12.6%). However, only two donors (0.09%) had granulocyte agglutinins without lymphocytotoxins. Although exclusion of HLA cross-reactivity in the sera containing both lymphocytotoxins and granulocyte agglutinins would have certainly detected more granulocyte antibodies, this would require absorption of the sera with pooled platelets and retesting for both HLA and granulocyte antibodies. However, we found it impractical to platelet-absorb large numbers of sera for this purpose.

In our experience, patients, especially mothers of infants affected by alloimmune neonatal neutropenia, are the best source of reagent-quality antisera. When a useful granulocyte antibody is detected in the serum of a patient, every effort should be made to persuade the patient to donate samples in the future or to undergo plasmapheresis if health permits. However, extended time and substantial referrals are necessary to acquire a variety of typing reagents by these means. Since random screening of donors and independent acquisition from clinical specimens are limited in producing reagent-quality antisera, it is often necessary to obtain typing reagents from other laboratories.

The American Red Cross Blood Services began a serum procurement and distribution service in 1981. The St. Paul Regional Red Cross Blood Services was appointed as the central Neutrophil Serology Reference Laboratory for the Blood Services, and was partially supported to attempt to find reagent-quality antisera for granulocyte serology. Red Cross Blood Services laboratories with referred patient samples believed to contain useful granulocyte antibodies available in sufficient quantities for reagent use were encouraged to send them to the central Neutrophil Serology Laboratory for (1) confirmation of the specificities; (2) absorption of the sera with pooled platelets to remove lymphocytotoxins if necessary; and (3) antibody characterization as to activity and working dilutions in various assays. The sera were then put in vials and lyophilized at the National Headquarters Reagent Production Laboratories. They are listed in a catalog and are available to all American Red Cross Blood Services Laboratories for use in typing granulocytes or establishing granulocyte antibody detection assays. They are also available to other investigators on an individually approved basis. Information may be obtained from Dr. John Lee or Larry Genkins, American Red Cross Blood Services, Reagent Production Laboratory, 4915 Auburn Avenue, Bethesda, MD 20814 (telephone (301) 652-4754).

Processing

Reagent antisera must be processed with extreme care to ensure correct classification of specificity. Failure to do so may perpetuate errors with repeated use in investigations and typing of antibody identification panel donors. We require that a minimum of 10 cells be tested, with at least two reactive and two nonreactive cells on the panel. This gives a P value of 0.022 and provides statistical assurance that the specificity is correctly assigned.

Antisera that are to be used as reagents are also tested by lymphocytotoxicity. Any reactivity is removed by absorption with purified pooled platelets. Reagents are also screened for red blood cell antibodies. In the rare cases in which they are detected, reactivity is removed by absorption with washed erythrocytes.

Antibodies are serially diluted in a buffer appropriate to the test assay to determine the maximum dilution still strongly reactive with the test cells with no changes in specificity. Use of a working dilution established in this way conserves valuable reagents.

Preservation

Reagent antisera may be stored frozen (see chapter 3) or lyophilized and stored at refrigerated temperatures (1° to 8°C) indefinitely. We have used lyophilized reagents for several years and find that they are convenient to use and easy to ship. No special storage facilities are required, and antibody activity is stabilized by minimizing repeated freezing and thawing. Despite the higher initial cost to prepare and process these reagents, they are an attractive alternative to freezing serum samples.

Chapter 13

Methods

The methods in this section are described as they are performed in our laboratory, except where another source is cited. We have attempted to include sufficient detail to permit performance of these procedures by those unfamiliar with granulocyte serologic techniques. References provide additional information on the development and/or applications of each method.

Standard equipment is used in many granulocyte serology assays. The following list is considered basic to the laboratory performing granulocyte testing. Equivalent instruments made by other manufacturers may be substituted as desired.

1. Refrigerated centrifuge with a horizontal rotor
2. Microcentrifuge
3. Adjustable micropipets (10 to 200 μL) and disposable tips
4. Microliter syringes and disposable tips (Hamilton)
   a. #705SN (needle point #3, 22 gauge)
   b. #1705 Tef LL with #31330 tip adaptor
   c. #83700 repeating dispenser
5. Repeating microliter dispenser with stream splitter
   a. Jet Pipet (#3202, York Instruments)
   b. Stream splitter (Robbins Scientific)
6. Dry-air incubator
7. −80°C freezer
8. Electronic cell counting apparatus or hemacytometer and microscope

9. pH meter

10. Balance

11. Vortex mixer

12. Glassware: beakers, flasks, serologic and transfer pipets, graduated cylinders, etc.

SECTION 1: Cell Preparation Techniques

1.1 Ficoll-Hypaque Gradients for Cell Isolation

Materials

1. Hydrometer for specific gravities 1.060 to 1.130 (Fisher Scientific)
2. 30 mL syringes (optional)
3. 3.5 inch, 17 gauge spinal needle (optional)
4. 17 × 120 mm polystyrene conical centrifuge tubes (15 mL)
5. Polystyrene culture tubes
   a. 16 × 150 mm
   b. 17 × 100 mm
6. Refrigerated centrifuge with a horizontal rotor

Reagents

1. Methyl cellulose
2. 0.9% saline solution
3. 75% Hypaque (Winthrop)
4. Ficoll 400 (Sigma)

Prepared Reagents

1. 1% methyl cellulose
   a. Prepare using 0.9% saline solution.
   b. Allow 18 to 24 hours for methyl cellulose to completely dissolve.
2. 33.9% Hypaque solution: Mix 50 mL 75% Hypaque with 60.5 mL distilled water.
3. 50% Hypaque solution: Mix 50 mL 75% Hypaque with 25 mL distilled water.
4. 9% Ficoll solution
   a. Dissolve 18 g of Ficoll in 200 mL distilled water.
   b. Maintain mixture at 4°C for 24 hours to completely dissolve the Ficoll.
5. Solution I (upper gradient fluid)
   a. Mix 31 mL 33.9% Hypaque with 69 mL 9% Ficoll.

    b. Adjust specific gravity to 1.080. If the solution is too heavy, add 9% Ficoll; if too light, add 33.9% Hypaque solution.

    c. Store the solution at 4°C; mix well before use.

6. Solution II (lower gradient fluid)

    a. Mix 37 mL 50% Hypaque with 63 mL 9% Ficoll.

    b. Adjust specific gravity to 1.120. If the solution is too heavy, add 9% Ficoll; if too light, add 50% Hypaque solution.

    c. Store at 4°C; mix well before use.

Method

1. Mix 10 mL fresh whole blood with an anticoagulant. The anticoagulant is determined by the assay in which the isolated cells are to be used.

2. Mix the anticoagulated blood with 2.5 mL 1% methyl cellulose in a 16 × 150 mm culture tube. Remove the tube cap, slant the tube at a 30° angle, and allow red blood cells to sediment for 20 minutes at room temperature (20°C to 24°C). This will leave a leukocyte-rich plasma (LRP).

    CAUTION: Allowing cells to sediment for more than 30 minutes will result in a reduced leukocyte yield.

3. Prepare the gradient tubes while the red blood cells are sedimenting. Place 3 mL Solution II in a conical centrifuge tube. Gently layer 3 mL of Solution I over Solution II with a transfer pipet. The two solutions must be at the same temperature. Maintain a smooth interface between the two solutions.

4. Remove the LRP from the culture tube and carefully layer up to 9 mL LRP over Solution I in the centrifuge tube.

5. *Alternate technique for steps 3 and 4*: Place up to 9 mL LRP in a conical centrifuge tube. Fill a syringe with Solution I and attach the spinal needle. Placing the needle tip at the bottom of the centrifuge tube, layer 3 mL Solution I under the LRP using slow, gentle pressure. Refill the syringe with Solution II and layer 3 mL under Solution I. This technique may be faster when processing large volumes of LRP.

6. Centrifuge the tube at 1,650 × g at 18°C for 15 minutes. Centrifugation produces three distinct layers:

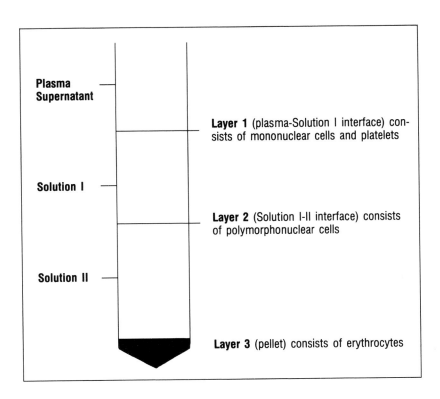

Plasma Supernatant

Layer 1 (plasma-Solution I interface) consists of mononuclear cells and platelets

Solution I

Layer 2 (Solution I-II interface) consists of polymorphonuclear cells

Solution II

Layer 3 (pellet) consists of erythrocytes

7. Wash leukocytes isolated from Layer 1 or Layer 2 twice in a 17 × 100 mm culture tube with 10 mL balanced salt solution or phosphate-buffered saline (PBS) solution before use.

Reference English D, Anderson BR: Single-step separation of red blood cells, granulocytes, and mononuclear leukocytes on discontinuous density gradients of Ficoll-Hypaque. *J Immunol Methods* 5:249–252, 1974.

1.2 Percoll Gradients for Cell Isolation

Materials
1. 30 mL syringes
2. 3.5 inch, 17 gauge spinal needle
3. Polystyrene culture tubes
   a. 16 × 150 mm
   b. 17 × 100 mm
4. Refrigerated centrifuge with a horizontal rotor

Reagents	1. Methyl cellulose
	2. 0.9% saline solution
	3. Sodium chloride (NaCl)
	4. Potassium chloride (KCl)
	5. Sodium phosphate, dibasic (Na_2HPO_4)
	6. Potassium phosphate, monobasic (KH_2PO_4)
	7. Percoll stock solution (Pharmacia)
	8. Sterile distilled water

Prepared Reagents

1. 1% methyl cellulose

    a. Prepare using 0.9% saline solution.

    b. Allow 18 to 24 hours for methyl cellulose to completely dissolve.

2. 10X Phosphate-buffered saline solution (PBS)

    a. Mix 80 g NaCl, 2 g KCl, 11.5 g Na_2HPO_4, and 2 g KH_2PO_4.

    b. Add sterile distilled water to make a total volume of 1,000 mL. Mix until dissolved.

    c. Adjust pH to 7.2.

    d. Pass through a 0.2 μm filter and store at 4°C in a sterile container. This reagent must be kept sterile.

3. PBS (1X): Dilute PBS (10X) 1:10 in sterile distilled water.

4. Percoll gradient solutions I and II

    a. Determine the volume of Percoll stock with the following equation:

    A = Volume of Percoll stock (mL)

    B = Volume needed of final working solution (mL)

    C = Density of desired working solution (Solution I = 1.075 g/mL; Solution II = 1.100 g/mL)

    D = Density of PBS (10X) solution = 1.065 g/mL

    E = Density of Percoll stock (stated on bottle)

$$A = B \times (C - \frac{(0.1 \times D - 0.9)}{E - 1.0}).$$

    b. Determine the volume of PBS (10X) as follows:

    0.1 × desired total volume (mL) of solution.

c. Mix the calculated volume of Percoll stock and PBS (10X). Dilute to final working volume with sterile water.

Example: To make 50 mL of Solution I (1.075 g/mL), using stock Percoll (1.129 g/mL)

$$A = 50 \times \frac{(1.075 - (0.1 \times 1.065) - 0.9)}{1.129 - 1.0}$$

$$= 26.6 \text{ mL stock Percoll}$$

22.6 mL stock Percoll
5.0 mL PBS (10X) : 0.1×50 mL final volume
22.4 mL Water
$\overline{50.0 \text{ mL Solution I}}$

d. Store in a sterile container at 4°C.

Method

1. Mix up to 50 mL fresh whole blood with an anticoagulant. The anticoagulant is determined by the assay in which the isolated cells are to be used.

2. Place 10 mL aliquots of anticoagulated blood into 16×150 mm culture tubes. Add 2.5 mL 1% methyl cellulose to each tube and mix. Remove the tube caps, slant the tubes at a 30° angle, and allow red blood cells to sediment for 20 minutes at room temperature (20°C to 24°C). This will leave a leukocyte-rich plasma (LRP).
   CAUTION: Allowing cells to sediment for more than 30 minutes will result in a reduced leukocyte yield.

3. Remove the LRP and place in 17×100 mm culture tubes. To concentrate, centrifuge at $400 \times g$ for 7 minutes. Combine cell pellets in a 17×100 mm culture tube and resuspend in 3 mL of PBS (1X).

4. Fill a syringe with Solution 1 and attach the spinal needle. Placing the needle tip at the bottom of the culture tube of LRP, layer 4 mL of Solution 1 under the LRP, using gentle, steady pressure. Refill the syringe with Solution 2 and layer 4 mL under Solution 1.

5. Centrifuge the tube at $400 \times g$ at 18°C for 20 minutes. Centrifugation produces three distinct layers:

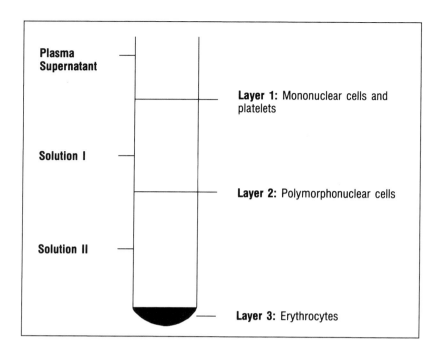

Plasma
Supernatant

Layer 1: Mononuclear cells and platelets

Solution I

Layer 2: Polymorphonuclear cells

Solution II

Layer 3: Erythrocytes

6. Wash leukocytes isolated from Layer 1 or Layer 2 twice in a 17 × 100 mm culture tube with 10 mL of a balanced salt solution or phosphate-buffered saline solution before use.

Reference   *Percoll: Methodology and Applications* (brochure). Piscataway, NJ, Pharmacia Fine Chemicals, 1982.

1.3 Preparation of Neutroplasts

Materials
1. 17 × 100 mm polystyrene culture tubes
2. Ultracentrifuge tubes
3. 30 mL syringes
4. 3.5 inch, 17 gauge spinal needle
5. Ultracentrifuge
6. Microscope slides and microscope

Reagents
1. 0.9% saline solution
2. Tromethamine (TRIS)

3. Sterile distilled water

4. Hydrochloric acid (HCl)

5. Ficoll-70 (Sigma)

6. Hepes powder

7. 10 N sodium hydroxide (NaOH)

8. 10X Hank's balanced salt solution (HBSS) (with calcium; without phenol red) (GIBCO)

9. Cytochalasin-B (Cyto-B)

10. Dimethyl sulfoxide (DMSO)

11. Ammonium chloride (NH_4Cl)

12. Potassium bicarbonate ($KHCO_3$)

13. 10% disodium edetate (Na_2EDTA)

14. Wright's stain

Prepared Reagents

1. 25 mM TRIS buffer
   a. Dissolve 3.03 g TRIS in 900 mL sterile water.
   b. Warm the solution to 37°C and adjust pH to 7.4 with HCl.
   c. Add sterile water to bring the volume to 1,000 mL. Pass through a 0.2 μm filter and store in a sterile bottle. Use only when sterile.

2. 40% Ficoll (stock)
   a. Dissolve 100 g Ficoll-70 in 200 mL 25 mM TRIS buffer. Stir overnight at 37°C to completely dissolve Ficoll.
   b. Add 25 mM TRIS buffer to bring the volume to 250 mL.
   c. Pass through a 0.45 μm filter. Store in a sterile bottle at 4°C. Use only if sterile.

3. 20X Hepes
   a. Dissolve 9.6 g Hepes in 100 mL sterile water.
   b. Adjust pH to 7.4 with 10N NaOH.
   c. Pass through a 0.2 μm filter. Store at 4°C.

4. Hank's balanced salt solution (HBSS)
   a. Mix 10 mL 10X HBSS and 5 mL 20X Hepes.
   b. Add sterile water to bring the volume to 100 mL. Adjust pH to 7.4.
   c. Pass through a 0.2 μm filter and store in a sterile bottle at 4°C.

5. Cytochalasin-B, stock (Cyto-B)
   a. Mix 10 mg Cyto-B and 1.0 mL DMSO.
   b. Store in a sterile, dark glass bottle at 20°C to 24°C.

6. Red Blood Cell (RBC) Lysing buffer

a. Mix 0.83 g NH$_4$Cl, 0.10 g KHCO$_3$, and 0.05 mL 10% Na$_2$ ETDA.

b. Add sterile water to bring the volume to 100 mL.

c. Pass through a 0.2 μm filter and store at 4°C.

7. Density gradients (prepare with sterile glassware and use sterile technique)

a. 25% Ficoll: Mix 75 mL 40% Ficoll and 45 mL HBSS. Store at 4°C.

b. 16% Ficoll: Mix 40 mL 40% Ficoll and 60 mL HBSS. Store at 4°C.

c. 12.5% Ficoll: Mix 25 mL 40% Ficoll and 55 mL HBSS. Store at 4°C.

Method

■ **Granulocyte Isolation**

1. Isolate the granulocytes from 200 to 250 mL sodium heparin anticoagulated blood (see procedure 1.1)

2. Discard the plasma supernatant and cells from Layer 1. Remove the polymorphonuclear leukocyte (PMN) layers (Layer 2) and place each in a 17 × 100 mm polystyrene culture tube. To each tube add 10 mL 0.9% saline solution and centrifuge at 400 × g at 18°C for 4 minutes. Decant the supernatants, resuspend the cell buttons, and pool into one tube. Wash again as above.

3. Decant the supernatant and resuspend cells in 1 mL RBC Lysing Buffer. Incubate in an ice bath for 5 minutes. Wash cells two times as above with 0.9% saline solution. If all red blood cells have not been lysed, repeat this lysing step. Incubating time may be increased to 10 minutes or 2 mL of RBC Lysing Buffer may be used if cell suspension is grossly contaminated with red blood cells after initial washes.

4. Add 5 mL HBSS to the final cell pellet. Count cells and then centrifuge at 400 × g for 4 minutes. Discard the supernatant.

■ **Test Procedure**

1. Incubate all tubes, reagents, rotor and carriers, syringe and spinal needle, and pipets at 37°C for a minimum of 1 hour, or preferrably overnight, before use. Add 5 μL of Cyto-B to 10 mL of each density gradient solution and mix vigorously immediately before incubation at 37°C.

CAUTION: All equipment *must* be maintained at 37°C during the procedure.

2. Resuspend cells in 4.5 mL 12.5% Ficoll-Cyto-B. Up to 4 × 10^8 cells can be placed on one gradient. If more cells are present,

resuspend in 9 mL 12.5% Ficoll-Cyto-B and divide equally between the two gradients. Incubate at 37°C for 10 to 15 minutes.

3. Transfer 4.5 mL of suspension to warmed ultracentrifuge tubes. Fill the syringe with attached spinal needle with 16% Ficoll-Cyto-B. Gently layer 5 mL 16% Ficoll-Cyto-B under the cell suspension, taking care to maintain a smooth interface.

4. Using the same technique, layer 5 mL 25% Ficoll-Cyto-B under the 16% Ficoll-Cyto-B.

5. Prepare a second gradient in the same way. If there is no second gradient, prepare a balance tube using 12.5% Ficoll without Cyto-B.

6. Balance the tubes and their carriers to within 0.5 grams. Carriers and rotor *must* be at 37°C. Centrifuge at 100,000 × g at 37°C for 30 minutes. Three distinct layers will appear:

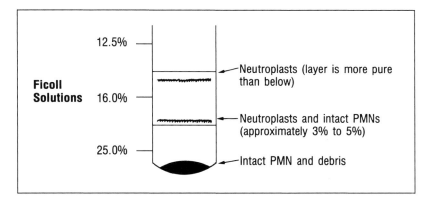

Harvest the neutroplast layers either separately or as one layer, depending upon purity desired.

7. Wash cytoplasts in HBSS, centrifuging for 15 minutes at 600 × g. The pellet should be very white.

8. Use Wright's stain to determine the purity of the preparation. Good preparations should contain less than 5% whole PMNs.

CAUTION: Neutroplasts are very fragile and can be lysed easily. When counting, lysing agents or white cell diluting fluids with acetic acid must not be used.

Reference   Roos D, Voetman AA, Meerhof LJ: Functional activity of enucleated human polymorphonuclear leukocytes. *J Cell Biol* 97:368–377, 1983.

1.4 Cryopreservation of Neutroplasts

Materials

1. 4.5 mL cryotubes
2. Water bath
3. Polystyrene box, walls 10 mm thick
4. 17 × 100 mm polystyrene culture tube
5. Centrifuge
6. −80° freezer

Reagents

1. Sodium chloride (NaCl)
2. Potassium chloride (KCl)
3. Sodium phosphate, dibasic (Na_2HPO_4)
4. Potassium phosphate, monobasic (KH_2PO_4)
5. Fetal calf serum
6. Dimethyl sulfoxide (DMSO)
7. Bovine serum albumin (BSA)
8. 1% paraformaldehyde (PFA)

Prepared Reagents

1. Incubation medium
   a. Dissolve 8.0 g NaCl, 0.2 g KCl, 1.15 g Na_2HPO_4, and 0.2 g KH_2PO_4 in 1,000 mL distilled water.
   b. Adjust pH to 7.2.
2. Suspension medium: 10% (v/v) fetal calf serum in incubation medium.
3. DMSO solution: 20% (v/v) dimethyl sulfoxide in suspension medium.
4. Wash solution: 0.5% bovine serum albumin in incubation medium.

Methods

■ *Freezing*

1. Suspend neutroplasts in 1 mL suspension medium in a 4.5 mL cryotube.
2. Cool suspended neutroplasts in the cryotube and a second tube containing 1 mL DMSO solution to 0°C in a water bath.
3. While maintaining 0°C temperature, add DMSO solution by drops to the neutroplast suspension, mixing continuously.

4. Place the cryotube containing the DMSO-neutroplasts mixture in a polystyrene box and freeze at −80°C.

■ Thawing

1. Cool 20 mL wash solution to 0°C in a water bath.

2. Place the cryotube with neutroplasts in a 37°C water bath until only a few ice crystals remain.

3. Transfer the suspension to a 17×100 mm polystyrene culture tube.

4. Add 10 mL precooled wash solution to the suspension in the culture tube. Centrifuge at $200 \times$ g for 10 minutes. Decant the supernatant and wash neutroplasts a second time.

5. Resuspend neutroplasts in a buffer suitable for the assay in which they are to be used. Neutroplasts may be counted as white cells on an electronic cell counter, but a lysing agent must not be added. Since neutroplast preparations contain few red blood cells, this causes no problem.

6. Fix neutroplasts with 1% PFA before use in the granulocyte immunofluorescence assay.

Reference   Voetman AA, Bot AAM, Roos D: Cryopreservation of enucleated human neutrophils (PMN cytoplasts). *Blood* 63:234–237, 1984.

SECTION 2: Antibody Detection Assays

2.1 Granulocyte Microagglutination Assay

Materials

1. Repeating microliter dispenser (York Instruments) with stream splitter
2. Microliter syringes with repeating dispensers (Hamilton)
   a. #1705 and disposable tips
   b. #705SN with needle
3. 60-well microtest tissue culture tray
4. 17 × 100 mm polystyrene culture tube
5. 1 mL microcentrifuge tubes
6. Microcentrifuge
7. Dry-air incubator
8. Inverted-phase microscope, with 6X phase objective and 12.5X widefield eyepiece
9. −80°C freezer

Reagents

1. Mineral oil, Saybolt viscosity 335/250
2. Sodium chloride (NaCl)
3. Potassium chloride (KCl)
4. Sodium phosphate, dibasic (Na_2HPO_4)
5. Potassium phosphate, monobasic (KH_2PO_4)
6. 22% bovine serum albumin (BSA)
7. 10% disodium edetate (Na_2EDTA)

Prepared Reagents

1. Phosphate-buffered saline solution (PBS)
   a. Dissolve 8.0 g NaCl, 0.2 g KCl, 1.15 g Na_2HPO_4, and 0.2 g KH_2PO_4 in 1,000 mL distilled water.
   b. Adjust pH to 7.2.
   c. Store at 4°C for up to 2 months. Examine for clarity before use.
2. Bovine serum albumin-EDTA solution (BSA-EDTA)

     a. Mix 15.0 mL 22% BSA, 4.4 mL 10% Na$_2$EDTA, and 90.6 mL PBS.

     b. Adjust pH to 7.2.

     c. Store at 4°C for up to 2 months. Examine for clarity before use.

3. Granulocyte resuspension solution (GRS)

     a. Mix 2.5 mL 22% BSA, 5.0 mL 10% Na$_2$EDTA, and 100 mL PBS.

     b. Adjust pH to 7.2.

     c. Store at 4°C for up to 2 months. Examine for clarity before use.

Method

■ Tray Preparation

1. Place 15 μL mineral oil in the appropriate wells of a microtest tissue culture tray using the microliter dispenser with stream splitter.

2. Prepare selected or serial dilutions of the test serum in BSA-EDTA (we routinely screen sera undiluted and diluted 1:4). Test all sera in duplicate.

3. Place 3 μL of each test serum and/or its corresponding dilution under the oil in the middle of each well with the microliter syringe and disposable tip.

4. Store the prepared tray at 4°C for use the same day, or at -80°C for longer periods.

■ Granulocyte Isolation

1. Isolate granulocytes from fresh whole blood anticoagulated with Na$_2$EDTA (see procedure 1.1).

2. Discard the plasma supernatant and cells from Layer 1. Remove the polymorphonuclear leukocyte (PMN) layer (Layer 2) and place in a 17 × 100 mm polystyrene culture tube.

3. Wash the cells twice with 10 mL PBS. Centrifuge at 300 × g at 18°C for 2 minutes for each wash. Decant supernatant and gently resuspend the cell pellet by manually rocking the tube.

4. Transfer the resuspended granulocyte pellet to a microcentrifuge tube. Add 1 mL BSA-EDTA. Centrifuge at 800 × g for 45 seconds.

5. Gently resuspend the cells in 1 mL GRS, using a transfer pipet and avoiding bubbles.

6. Count cells and adjust to 5 × 10^6/mL in GRS.

■ Test Procedure

1. Thaw the antisera tray 15 minutes before use. Remove the tray cover.

2. Thoroughly resuspend the granulocyte suspension using a transfer pipet.

3. Add 1 μL of the cell suspension to the serum in the bottom of each well using a microliter syringe with needle. Wipe the tip and expel 1 drop of cells between different antisera to prevent cross-contamination. Rinse the syringe in saline solution when changing granulocyte suspensions and in distilled water after use.

4. Replace the tray cover and incubate at 30°C in a dry-air incubator for 5 to 6 hours.

Interpretation of Results

Read the results on an inverted phase microscope. The strength of the reaction is graded from 0 to 4+ according to the proportion of cells participating in the reaction.

Percentage of Agglutination	Grade
Greater than 90%	4+
50% to 89%	3+
25% to 49%	2+
Less than 25%	1+
None	0

Individual cells can be discerned in true agglutinates. Careful examination will reduce the possibility of debris, possibly with adherent cells, being interpreted as agglutinates.

Occasional sera (ie, from patients on chemotherapy) may be cytotoxic to granulocytes. These nonviable cells appear dark rather than refractile microscopically. Such sera, especially undiluted, cannot be evaluated in the granulocyte agglutination assay as cell viability is necessary for agglutination to occur.

Grossly-hemolyzed or bacterially-contaminated sera may cause false-positive reactions.

References

Lalezari P, Jiang A, Lee S: A microagglutination technique for detection of leukocyte agglutinins, in Ray JG, Hare DB, Pederson PD, et al (eds): National Institute of Allergy and Infectious Disease Manual: *A Tissue Typing Technique.* U.S. Department of Health Education and Welfare publication No. (NIH)77-545, pp 4–6, 1976.

Lalezari P, Pryce SC: Detection of neutrophil and platelet antibodies in immunologically induced neutropenia and thrombocytopenia, in Rose

NR, Friedmann H (eds). *Manual of clinical immunology.* Washington, DC, American Society for Microbiology, pp 744–749, 1980.

2.2 Microgranulocyte Cytotoxicity Assay

Materials

1. Micropore filters
   a. 0.45 μm
   b. 0.20 μm
2. 10 mL sterile culture tubes or bottles, with caps
3. 17 × 100 mm polystyrene culture tube
4. 1 mL microcentrifuge tubes
5. Microcentrifuge
6. Repeating microliter dispensers (York Instruments) with stream splitters
7. Microliter syringes with repeating dispensers (Hamilton)
   a. #1710 and disposable tips
   b. #1725 and disposable tips
   c. #705SN with needle
8. 60-well microtest tissue culture tray
9. Vortex mixer
10. Hot plate
11. 50 × 75 mm coverglasses
12. Inverted phase microscope, with 6X phase objective and 12.5X widefield eyepiece
13. −80°C freezer

Reagents

1. Mineral oil, Saybolt viscosity 335/250
2. Hank's 10X balanced salt solution (HBSS) containing Ca^{2+} and Mg^{2+} (Gibco)
3. McCoy's 5a medium (Gibco)
4. Fetal calf serum
5. Hepes powder
6. 10 N sodium hydroxide, (NaOH)
7. 95% ethanol
8. Benzyl alcohol

9. Eosin-y

10. 0.5% phenol red

11. 37% formaldehyde, reagent grade

12. Potassium hydroxide (KOH)

13. Rabbit complement, mature pooled (Gibco)

14. Petrolatum

15. Sterile water

16. Acid citrate dextrose (ACD)

Prepared Reagents

1. Hank's balanced salt solution (HBSS)

   a. Mix 10 mL Hank's 10X solution with 90 mL sterile water.

   b. Adjust pH to 6.8.

   c. Shake well and pass through a 0.20 μm filter.

   d. Put 5 to 10 mL aliquots in sterile culture tubes or bottles. Store at 4°C. Observe for fungal contamination and/or color change before use.

2. Hepes buffer

   a. Dissolve 23.8 g Hepes powder in 75 mL sterile water. Add sterile water to a total volume of 100 mL.

   b. Adjust the pH to 6.8 using 10N NaOH.
      CAUTION: Do not exceed the 6.8 reading as HCl cannot be used to lower pH, and the solution must be discarded.

   c. Pass through a 0.20 μm filter. Place 10 mL aliquots in sterile culture tubes or bottles. Store at 4°C.

3. Fetal calf serum (FCS)

   a. Defrost a bottle of FCS in *cold* water.
      CAUTION: Warm or hot water or shaking will denature the protein.

   b. Mix FCS gently and pass through a 0.45 μm filter. Divide into aliquots and store at −80°C.

4. McCoy's solution

   a. Mix 1.2 g McCoy's 5a medium, 0.6 mL fetal calf serum, 0.7 mL 0.5% phenol red, and 1 mL Hepes buffer. Add sterile water to make a final volume of 100 mL.

   b. Adjust pH to 6.8.

   c. Mix gently and pass through a 0.20 μm filter.

   d. Place 10 mL aliquots in sterile culture tubes or bottles. Store at 4°C.

5. Alcohol-McCoy's solution

a. Add one part benzyl alcohol to nine parts 95% ethanol. This mixture must be clear.

b. Dilute the alcohol solution 1:50 in McCoy's solution.

c. Prepare daily immediately before use.

6. Rabbit complement: Complement activity can vary from lot to lot and among manufacturers. In addition, normal rabbit serum can cause non-specific lysis of human granulocytes. Initially, complement should be used as provided by the manufacturer. If granulocyte toxicity is observed, the toxic factor can be removed by absorption with a pool of human red blood cells.

a. Absorb complement with packed washed red blood cells (9:1 v/v) for 30 minutes at 0°C.

b. Repeat the absorption a second time using a fresh pool of packed red blood cells.

c. Centrifuge absorbed rabbit serum at $1,000 \times$ g at 4°C for 5 minutes to remove red blood cells. Complement *must* be free of all red blood cells prior to use.

d. Store small aliquots at -80°C. Thaw immediately before use. Complement activity is best maintained at cool temperatures. Prepared aliquots of frozen complement should only be thawed once prior to use.

7. 8% eosin: Filter daily before use.

8. Formaldehyde solution

a. Add 0.5 mL 0.5% phenol red to 125 mL formaldehyde.

b. Add concentrated KOH by drops until the solution is a salmon color (pH 7.0 to 7.2).

c. Prepare daily immediately before use.

Method

■ *Tray Preparation*

1. Place 5 μL of mineral oil in the appropriate wells of a microtest tissue culture tray, using a microliter dispenser with stream splitter.

2. If desired, prepare a selected dilution of the test serum in McCoy's solution (we normally test sera undiluted). Test all sera in triplicate.

3. Place 2 μL of each test serum and/or its corresponding dilution under the oil in the middle of each well, using a microliter syringe (#1710) and disposable tips.

4. Store the prepared tray at 4°C for use the same day, or at -80°C for longer periods.

■ Granulocyte Isolation

1. Isolate granulocytes from fresh whole blood anticoagulated with ACD, using 1.5 mL ACD per 10 mL whole blood (see procedure 1.1).

2. Discard the plasma supernatant and cells from Layer 1. Remove the polymorphonuclear leukocyte (PMN) layer (Layer 2) and place in a 17×100 mm polystyrene culture tube.

3. Wash the cells twice with 10 mL Hank's solution. Centrifuge at $300 \times$ g at 18°C for 2 minutes for each wash. Decant supernatant and gently resuspend the cell pellet by manually rocking the tube.

4. Transfer the resuspended granulocyte pellet to a microcentrifuge tube. Add 1 mL McCoy's solution. Centrifuge at $800 \times$ g for 45 seconds. The cells must be maintained in this solution until immediately before use.

5. Gently resuspend the cells in 1 mL alcohol-McCoy's solution.

6. Count cells and adjust the concentration to 6 to 8×10^6/mL in alcohol-McCoy's solution.

■ Test Procedure

1. Thaw the antisera tray 15 minutes before use.

2. Thoroughly resuspend the granulocyte suspension using a transfer pipet.

3. Add 1 μL of the granulocyte suspension to the serum under oil in each well using a microliter syringe with needle (#705SN). Wipe the tip and expel 1 drop of cells between different antisera to prevent cross-contamination. Rinse the syringe in saline solution when changing granulocyte suspensions, and in distilled water after use.

4. Mix by pressing the edge of the tray against the vibrating head of a vortex mixer for a few seconds.

5. Incubate the tray for 45 minutes at selected sensitization temperatures. We incubate at room temperature (20°C to 24°C) and 37°C.

6. Add 5 μL of rabbit complement to the cell-serum mixture under the oil using a microliter syringe (#1725) and disposable tip.

7. Incubate at room temperature for 3 hours.

8. Add 5 μL 8% eosin to the cell-serum-complement mixture under the oil using a microliter syringe (#1725) with disposable tip. Wait 10 minutes for dye penetration.

9. Add 10 μL of formaldehyde solution under the oil in each well, using a microliter dispenser with stream splitter.

10. Lower a 50 × 75 mm coverglass onto the wells of the tray flattening the top of the droplets.

11. Heat petrolatum on a hot plate until it is liquid. Dispense petrolatum around the edges of the coverglass with a transfer pipet, sealing it to prevent evaporation and siphoning of fluid from individual wells.

12. Allow the tray to sit undisturbed for approximately 30 minutes until the granulocytes have settled. Read the results or store overnight at 4°C and read the next day.

Interpretation of Results

Read the reactions with an inverted-phase contrast microscope. Intact granulocytes are small and refractile, while lysed granulocytes are larger and stained dark with eosin. Good phase contrast is necessary for definitive differentiation of cells with and without intact membranes.

The principle in reading is to establish the proportion of intact granulocytes in the negative control as the baseline. Lysed cells in negative controls are not due to antibody reaction, but are background that must be considered when reading other reactions.

Score the reaction according to the proportion of granulocytes which have been lysed.

Scoring Code	% Lysed Cells	Interpretation
1	0% to 10%	Negative
2	11% to 20%	Negative
4	21% to 35%	Questionable positive
5	36% to 50%	Weak positive
6	51% to 80%	Positive
8	81% to 100%	Strong positive

References

Hasegawa T, Graw RG, Terasaki PI: A microgranulocyte cytotoxicity test. *Transplantation* 15:492–498, 1973.

Drew SI, Bergh O, McClelland J, et al: Antigenic specificities detected on papainized human granulocytes by microgranulocytotoxicity. *Transplant Proc* 9:639–645, 1977.

Drew SI, Carter BM, Guidera D, et al: Further aspects of microgranulocytotoxicity. *Transfusion* 19:434–443, 1979.

2.3 Double Fluorochromatic Microgranulocyte Cytotoxicity Assay

Materials

1. Microliter syringes with repeating dispensers (Hamilton)
   a. #1705 with disposable tips
   b. #1725 with disposable tips
   c. #705SN with needle
2. Repeating microliter dispenser (York Instruments) and stream splitter
3. 60-well microtest tissue culture tray
4. 17 × 100 mm polystyrene culture tube
5. 1 mL microcentrifuge tubes
6. Microcentrifuge
7. Fluorescence microscope (inverted preferred), equipped with excitation and barrier filters to permit simultaneous visualization of green and red fluorescence
8. −80°C freezer
9. 0.2 μm micropore filter

Reagents

1. Mineral oil, Saybolt viscosity 335/250
2. Sodium chloride (NaCl)
3. Potassium chloride (KCl)
4. Sodium phosphate, dibasic (Na_2HPO_4)
5. Potassium phosphate, monobasic (KH_2PO_4)
6. Hepes powder
7. 10 N sodium hydroxide (NaOH)
8. Hank's 10X balanced salt solution (HBSS) containing Ca^{2+} and Mg^{2+} (Gibco)
9. Bovine serum albumin (BSA)
10. Fluorescein diacetate (FDA) (Fisher Scientific)
11. Dimethyl sulfoxide (DMSO)
12. Rabbit complement, mature pooled (Gibco)
13. Ethidium bromide
14. Disodium edetate (Na_2EDTA)
15. Sterile distilled water
16. Acid citrate dextrose (ACD)

1. Phosphate-buffered saline solution (PBS)

    a. Dissolve 8.00 g NaCl, 0.20 g KCl, 1.15 g Na_2HPO_4, and 0.20 g KH_2PO_4 in 1,000 mL distilled water.

    b. Adjust pH to 7.2.

2. 0.2% bovine serum albumin in PBS (PBS-BSA)

3. 20X Hepes

    a. Dissolve 9.6 g Hepes powder in 100 mL sterile water.

    b. Adjust pH to 7.2 with 10 N NaOH.

    c. Pass through 0.2 μm filter; store in sterile bottle at 4°C.

4. Hank's balanced salt solution (HBSS)

    a. Mix 10 mL 10X Hank's and 5 mL 20X Hepes.

    b. Bring the volume to 100 mL with sterile water. Adjust pH to 7.2

    c. Pass through a 0.2 μm filter and store at 4°C.

5. Rabbit complement: Complement activity can vary from lot to lot and among manufacturers. In addition, normal rabbit serum can cause nonspecific lysis of human granulocytes. Initially complement should be used as provided by the manufacturer. If granulocyte toxicity is observed, the toxic factor can be removed by absorption with a pool of human red blood cells.

    a. Absorb complement with packed washed red blood cells (9:1 v/v) for 30 minutes at 0°C.

    b. Repeat the absorption a second time using a fresh pool of packed red blood cells.

    c. Centrifuge absorbed rabbit serum at 1,000 × g at 4°C for 5 minutes to remove red blood cells. Complement *must* be free of all red blood cells prior to use.

    d. Store small aliquots at −80°C. Thaw immediately before use.

    NOTE: Complement activity is best maintained at cool temperatures. Prepared aliquots of frozen complement should only be thawed once prior to use.

6. Fluorescein diacetate (FDA): Mix 100 mg FDA in 10 mL DMSO. Store in the dark at room temperature.

7. Ethidium bromide

    a. Stock solution: Dissolve 1 mg ethidium bromide in 10 mL 5% Na_2EDTA. Freeze 1 mL aliquots at −80°C, keeping 1 aliquot at 4°C in darkness for daily use.

b. Working solution: Dilute the stock solution 1:4 in 1.25% Na_2EDTA in HBSS prior to use.

| Method | ■ **Tray Preparation** |

Method

■ *Tray Preparation*

1. Place 5 μL of mineral oil in the appropriate wells of a microtest tissue culture tray using a repeating microliter dispenser with stream splitter.

2. If desired, prepare a selected dilution of the test serum in HBSS (we normally test sera undiluted in triplicate).

3. Place 1 μL of each test serum and/or its corresponding dilution under the oil in the middle of each well using a microliter syringe (#1705) and disposable tips.

4. Store the tray at 4°C for use the same day, or at -80°C for longer periods.

■ *Granulocyte Isolation*

1. Isolate the granulocytes from fresh whole blood anticoagulated with ACD using 1.5 mL ACD per 10 mL blood (see procedure 1.1).

2. Discard the plasma supernatant and cells from Layer 1. Remove the polymorphonuclear leukocyte (PMN) layer (Layer 2) and place in a 17 × 100 mm polystyrene culture tube.

3. Wash the cells twice with 10 mL PBS-BSA solution. Centrifuge for each wash at 300 × g at 18°C for 5 minutes. Discard the supernatant. Gently resuspend the cell pellet by manually rocking the tube.

4. Resuspend the cells in PBS-BSA. Count and adjust the concentration to 5 × 10^6/mL.

5. Label the cells by adding 2 μL of FDA solution to each mL of granulocytes. Mix well. Incubate at 20°C to 24°C for 5 minutes in the dark.

6. Wash the cells twice more with PBS-BSA as in step 3.

7. Resuspend the cells in HBSS. Count and adjust the concentration to 5.0 × 10^6/mL.

■ *Test Procedure*

1. Thaw the antisera tray 15 minutes before use.

2. Thoroughly resuspend the granulocyte suspension using a transfer pipet.

3. Add 1 μL of the granulocyte suspension to the serum under oil in each well.

4. Centrifuge the tray at 300 × g for 5 minutes to mix the serum and cells.

5. Incubate at 20°C for 60 minutes.

6. Add 5 μl of rabbit complement to each well with a microliter syringe (#1725) and disposable tip.

7. Incubate at 20°C for 90 to 120 minutes in the dark.

8. Add 2 μL of freshly prepared ethidium bromide working solution to each well. Allow 10 minutes for staining of dead cells to occur.

9. Fill the wells to roundness with PBS-BSA and wait 5 minutes for disturbed cells to settle. Remove the excess ethidium bromide by aspiration or flicking. This step may have to be repeated if intense red fluorescence remains in the fluid.

10. Centrifuge the tray at 500 × g for 5 minutes to bed cells before reading.

Interpretation of Results

Read the reactions within 2 hours using a fluorescence microscope. Viable granulocytes appear as bright green fluorescing cells. The nonviable (reactive) cells take up ethidium bromide, a red dye preferential to dead cell nuclei.

The principle in reading is to establish the proportion of viable granulocytes in the negative control as the baseline. Nonviable cells in negative controls are usually not due to antibody reaction, but are merely a background which must be considered when reading other reactions.

Score the reactions according to the proportion of dead cells.

Scoring Code	% Dead Cells	Interpretation
1	0% to 10%	Negative
2	11% to 20%	Negative
4	21% to 40%	Weak or questionable positive
6	41% to 80%	Positive
8	81% to 100%	Strong positive

References

Thompson JS, Severson CD: Granulocyte antigens, in Bell CA (ed): *A seminar on antigens on blood cells and body fluid.* Washington, DC, American Association of Blood Banks, pp 151–187, 1980.

Thompson JS, Overlin VL, Herbick JM, et al: New granulocyte antigens demonstrated by microgranulocytotoxicity assay. *J Clin Invest* 65:143–149, 1980.

Thompson JS, Overlin V, Severson CD, et al: Demonstration of granulocyte, monocyte and endothelial cell antigens by double fluorochromatic microcytotoxicity testing. *Transplant Proc* 12:1, pp 26–31, 1980.

2.4 Granulocyte Immunofluorescence Assays

2.4–A   Micro Method: Indirect and Direct Testing

Materials	1. Adjustable micropipet (10 to 200 μL) and disposable tips
	2. Polystyrene U-bottom microtiter tray and sealer
	3. 17 × 100 mm polystyrene culture tube
	4. Repeating microliter dispenser (York Instruments) with stream splitter
	5. Centrifuge with horizontal rotor
	6. 8 mm printed microscope slides, heavy teflon-coated (Cel-Line Associates)
	7. 24 × 60 mm coverglasses, No. 1
	8. Microliter syringe #1705 and disposable tips (Hamilton)
	9. Reflected light fluorescence microscope with FITC filtration system (excitation filter: 450 to 490 nm, dichroic mirror: 510 nm, barrier filter: 515 nm). Objective: 40 × dry N.A. 0.75
	10. −80°C freezer
	11. Dry-air incubator

Reagents	1. Sodium chloride (NaCl)
	2. Sodium phosphate, monobasic (NaH$_2$PO$_4 \cdot$H$_2$O)
	3. Sodium phosphate, dibasic (Na$_2$HPO$_4$)
	4. Bovine serum albumin (BSA)
	5. Ammonium chloride (NH$_4$Cl)
	6. Potassium bicarbonate (KHCO$_3$)
	7. 10% disodium edetate (Na$_2$EDTA)
	8. Paraformaldehyde (PFA)
	9. 1N hydrochloric acid (HCl)
	10. Fluorescein-conjugated goat antiserum to human immunoglobulins—F(ab')$_2$ fragments (Kallestad):
	a. Total Ig (#141)
	b. IgG (#139)
	c. IgM (#140)
	d. IgA (#137)
	11. Glycerol

Prepared Reagents

1. Phosphate-buffered saline solution (PBS)

   a. Dissolve 8.2 g NaCl, 0.142 g $NaH_2PO_4 \cdot H_2O$, and 1.38 g Na_2HPO_4 in 1,000 mL distilled water.

   b. Adjust pH to 7.0.

2. 0.2% bovine serum albumin in PBS (PBS-BSA): Prepare fresh weekly.

3. NH_4Cl solution: Dissolve 0.83 g NH_4Cl and 0.10 g $KHCO_3$ in 100 mL distilled water. Add 0.05 mL 10% Na_2EDTA.

4. Paraformaldehyde (PFA)

   a. 4% stock solution: Dissolve 4 g PFA in 100 mL PBS by heating to 70°C. (CAUTION: Container should be covered during heating to restrict fumes.) Adjust pH to 7.0 to 7.2 with 1 N HCl. Store at 4°C to 6°C in darkness for up to 3 months.

   b. 1% working solution: Dilute stock solution 1:4 in PBS. Store at 4°C to 6°C in darkness for up to 2 weeks.

5. Fluorescein-conjugated goat antiserum to human immunoglobulin (FITC-AHG): Dilute antiglobulin serum in PBS immediately before use. The dilution should allow maximal specific fluorescence with minimal background fluorescence. Determine the dilution for each lot by checkerboard titrations, using dilutions (ie, 1:1, 1:5, 1:10, etc.) of a known positive serum and negative serum against dilutions (ie, 1:50, 1:75, 1:100, 1:125, 1:150, etc.) of antiglobulin serum. Select the dilution of antiglobulin serum which yields the strongest fluorescence with the positive serum, while showing no fluorescence with the negative serum.

6. Glycerol—PBS: Dilute glycerol in PBS (3:1, v/v).

Method

■ **Tray Preparation**

1. Pipet 20 μL of each undilute serum into a well of a microtiter tray using a micropipet and disposable tips. Make serial or selected dilutions in the wells using PBS-BSA as diluent (ie, 1:5 dilution = 5 μL serum and 15 μL PBS-BSA). (We routinely screen sera undiluted and at a 1:5 dilution.)

2. Cover the tray with a sealer. Store tray at 4°C to 6°C when testing is to be done within 24 to 48 hours. For delayed testing, freeze the tray at −80°C.

■ **Granulocyte Isolation**

1. Isolate granulocytes from fresh whole blood anticoagulated with Na_2EDTA (see procedure 1.1).

Use the following guidelines to determine the required blood volume when testing patients' granulocytes (sufficient cells may be obtained from smaller volumes):

Absolute Neutrophil Count/μL	Required Blood Volume (mL)
Greater than 2,000	15
1,000 to 2,000	20 to 30
Less than 1,000	30 or more*

*Obtaining sufficient granulocytes for testing at this level may be difficult. When limited numbers of cells are obtained, testing may be done with a cell suspension of as few as 3×10^6/mL granulocytes.

2. Discard the plasma supernatant and cells from Layer 1. Remove the polymorphonuclear leukocyte (PMN) layer (Layer 2) and place in a 17×100 mm polystyrene culture tube.

3. Wash the cells twice with 10 mL of PBS-BSA. Centrifuge at $300 \times$ g for 2 minutes each time. Decant the supernatant. Gently resuspend the cell button by manually rocking the tube. If the cell pellet appears pink (red blood cells present), proceed with lysing, step 4. If red blood cells are not visible, continue with step 5.

4. To lyse red blood cells, add 1 mL cold NH_4Cl solution to the resuspended granulocyte pellet. Incubate for 5 minutes on ice. Wash cells twice with 10 mL PBS-BSA, centrifuging at $300 \times$ g for 2 minutes each time. Repeat this step as necessary until red blood cells are no longer visible.

5. Add 2 mL 1% PFA to the resuspended granulocytes, and mix gently. Incubate for 5 minutes at 20°C to 24°C.

6. Wash cells 2 more times, as in step 3. Gently resuspend the cells in 1 mL PBS-BSA.

7. Count the cells and adjust the concentration to 10 to 12×10^6/mL in PBS-BSA.

■ *Test Procedure: Indirect Granulocyte Immunofluorescence*

1. If frozen, thaw the antisera tray 15 minutes before use. Allow the tray to reach room temperature before removing the sealer.

2. Thoroughly resuspend granulocytes using a transfer pipet and avoiding bubbles.

3. Add 20 μL of the granulocyte suspension to each well containing serum using a micropipet. Gently tap plates on a flat surface to mix cells and sera.

4. Incubate uncovered plates at 37°C for 30 minutes in a dry-air incubator.

5. Add 200 μL PBS-BSA to each well using a microliter dispenser with stream splitter. (CAUTION: Position the stream splitter carefully to avoid cross-contamination of wells.) Centrifuge at 200 × g for 1 minute. Decant supernatant by vigorously flicking the tray. While inverted, blot the tray on absorbent gauze. Repeat twice more.

6. To each well, add 20 μL of an appropriate dilution of FITC-AHG using a micropipet (we use FITC-AHG to total immunoglobulins for routine screening of sera). Mix by gently rocking the tray.

7. Incubate plates at 20°C to 24°C for 30 minutes in the dark.

8. Wash cells 3 times as in step 5.

9. Add 10 μL of glycerol-PBS to each well using a micropipet. Gently tap the tray on a flat surface to mix the glycerol-PBS with the cells.

10. Gently resuspend cells using a microliter syringe and disposable tip. Transfer 2 to 3 μL cell suspension to a clean printed microscope slide. Apply a coverglass and allow cells to settle in the dark for a minimum of 15 minutes before reading.

■ **Test Procedure: Direct Granulocyte Immunofluorescence**

1. If frozen, thaw the antisera tray 15 minutes before use. Allow the tray to reach room temperature before removing the sealer.

2. Thoroughly resuspend granulocytes using a transfer pipet and avoiding bubbles.

3. Add 20 μL of the granulocyte suspension to each well containing serum using a micropipet. Gently tap plates on a flat surface to mix cells and sera.

4. Incubate uncovered plates at 37°C for 30 minutes in a dry-air incubator.

5. Add 200 μL PBS-BSA to each well using a microliter dispenser with stream splitter. (CAUTION: Position the stream splitter carefully to avoid cross contamination of wells.) Centrifuge at 200 × g for 1 minute. Decant supernatant by vigorously flicking the tray. While inverted, blot the tray on absorbent gauze. Repeat once more.

6. Add 20 μL cell suspension to empty wells for direct testing. Wash all cells one more time, as in step 5.

7. Add 20 μL of appropriate dilutions of FITC-AHG to each well (we use FITC-AHG to total immunoglobulins, IgG, IgM, and IgA for direct testing when sufficient granulocytes can be isolated). Mix by gently rocking the tray.

8. Incubate plates at 20°C to 24°C for 30 minutes in the dark.

9. Wash cells three times, as in step 5.

10. Add 10 µL of glycerol-PBS to each well using a micropipet. Gently tap the tray on a flat surface to mix the glycerol-PBS with the cells.

11. Gently resuspend cells using a microliter syringe and disposable tip. Transfer 2 to 3 µL cell suspension to a clean printed microscope slide. Apply a coverglass and allow cells to settle in the dark for a minimum of 15 minutes before reading.

Interpretation of Results

Read the slides using a fluorescence microscope. The strengths of the reactions are graded 0 to 4 according to the characteristics of fluorescent staining.

Grade	Characteristic
0	No cell-bound fluorescence
±	Minimal cell-bound fluorescence
1	Fluorescent dots barely outline cell membrane distinctly
2	Fluorescence appears as closely-spaced but distinct dots on cell membrane
3	Fluorescent dots on cell membrane are partially merged to form bands
4	Fluorescence appears as solid ring around cell

Although minimized by the PFA-fixation of granulocytes and use of $F(ab')_2$ fragments of antihuman globulin, some non-specific binding of immunoglobulins may still occur. Negative or 1+ reactions are acceptable for negative controls. Reactivity of negative controls must be used as the baseline for interpretation of other reactions with any panel cell.

Gentle handling is required to prevent damage to the granulocyte membranes. When damaged, cells will have cytoplasmic rather than membrane fluorescence and cannot be evaluated.

Positive reactions due to binding of immune complexes are not visually distinguishable from those caused by antibodies. Immune complexes may be excluded only when polymorphism is evident.

Normal donor cells may be tested in parallel with patients' cells to verify accurate dilutions of the conjugates in direct testing. They should demonstrate the appropriate reactions with positive and negative control sera, and direct testing of normal donor cells should be negative.

References

Lalezari P, Pryce SC: Detection of neutrophil and platelet antibodies in immunologically induced neutropenia and thrombocytopenia, in Rose NR, Friedmann H (eds): *Manual of clinical immunology.* Washington, DC, American Society for Microbiology, pp 744–749, 1980.

Verheugt FWA, von dem Borne AEGKr, Decary S, et al: The detection of granulocyte alloantibodies with an indirect immunofluorescence test. *Brit J Haematol* 36:533–544, 1977.

Press C, Kline WE, Clay ME, et al: A microtiter modification of granulocyte immunofluorescence. *Vox Sang* 49:110–113, 1985.

2.4–B   Tube Method: Indirect and Direct Testing

NOTE: Although more cumbersome, the tube method may be necessary to prepare granulocytes in sufficient quantities for testing in flow cytofluorometry or electron microscopy.

Materials

1. Adjustable micropipet (10 to 200 μL) and disposable tips
2. 1 mL microcentrifuge tubes and stoppers
3. −80°C freezer
4. 17 × 100 mm polystyrene culture tube
5. Centrifuge with horizontal rotor
6. 60 mL syringe
7. Microcentrifuge
8. 8 mm printed microscope slides, heavy teflon-coated (Cel-Line Associates)
9. 24 × 60 mm coverglasses, No. 1
10. Reflected light fluorescence microscope with FITC filtration system (excitation filter: 450 to 490 nm, dichroic mirror: 510 nm, barrier filter: 515 nm). Objective: 40 × dry N.A. 0.75
11. Dry-air incubator
12. Vortex mixer

Reagents

1. Sodium chloride (NaCl)
2. Sodium phosphate, monobasic ($NaH_2PO_4 \cdot H_2O$)
3. Sodium phosphate, dibasic (Na_2HPO_4)
4. Bovine serum albumin (BSA)
5. Ammonium chloride (NH_4Cl)
6. Potassium carbonate ($KHCO_3$)
7. 10% disodium edetate (Na_2EDTA)
8. Paraformaldehyde (PFA)
9. 1 N hydrochloric acid (HCl)
10. Fluorescein-conjugated goat antiserum to human immuno-globulins—$F(ab')_2$ fragments (Kallestad):
    a. Total Ig (#141)

          b. IgG (#139)

          c. IgM (#140)

          d. IgA (#137)

    11. Glycerol

Prepared Reagents

1. Phosphate-buffered saline solution (PBS)

    a. Dissolve 8.2 g NaCl, 0.142 g $NaH_2PO_4 \cdot H_2O$, and 1.38 g Na_2HPO_4 in 1,000 mL distilled water.

    b. Adjust pH to 7.0

2. 0.2% bovine serum albumin in PBS (PBS-BSA): Prepare fresh weekly.

3. NH_4Cl solution: Dissolve 0.83 g NH_4Cl and 0.10 g $KHCO_3$ in 100 mL distilled water. Add 0.05 mL 10% NA_2EDTA.

4. Paraformaldehyde (PFA)

    a. 4% stock solution: Dissolve 4 g PFA in 100 mL PBS by heating to 70°C. (CAUTION: Container should be covered during heating to restrict fumes.) Adjust pH to 7.0 to 7.2 with 1 N HCl. Store at 4°C to 6°C in darkness for up to 3 months.

    b. 1% working solution: Dilute stock solution 1:4 in PBS. Store at 4°C to 6°C in darkness for up to 2 weeks.

5. Fluorescein-conjugated goat antiserum to human immunoglobulin (FITC-AHG): Dilute antiglobulin serum in PBS immediately before use. The dilution should allow maximal specific fluorescence with minimal background fluorescence. Determine the dilution for each lot by checkerboard titrations, using dilutions (ie, 1:1, 1:5, 1:10, etc.) of a known positive serum and negative serum against dilutions (ie, 1:50, 1:75, 1:100, 1:125, 1:150, etc.) of antiglobulin serum. Select the dilution of antiglobulin serum which yields the strongest fluorescence with the positive serum, while showing no fluorescence with the negative serum.

    NOTE: The optimal dilution of FITC-AHG must be determined by the above procedure using the method (micro or tube) in which it is to be used. The tube method usually requires a lesser dilution of FITC-AHG.

6. Glycerol—PBS: Dilute glycerol in PBS (3:1, v/v).

Method

■ Tube Preparation

1. Pipet 40 μL of each undilute serum into a microcentrifuge tube using a micropipet and disposable tips. Make serial or selected dilutions using PBS-BSA as diluent. (We routinely screen sera undiluted and at a 1:5 dilution.)

2. Seal the tubes with stoppers.

3. Store the tubes at 4°C to 6°C when testing is to be done within 24 to 48 hours. For delayed testing, freeze the tubes at −80°C.

■ Granulocyte Isolation

1. Isolate granulocytes from fresh whole blood anticoagulated with Na_2EDTA (see procedure 1.1).

Use the following guidelines to determine the required blood volume when testing patients' granulocytes (sufficient cells may be obtained from smaller volumes):

Absolute Neutrophil Count/μL	Required Blood Volume (mL)
Greater than 2,000	15
1,000 to 2,000	20 to 30
Less than 1,000	30 or more*

* Obtaining sufficient granulocytes for testing at this level may be difficult. When limited numbers of cells are obtained, testing may be done with a cell suspension of as few as 3×10^6/mL granulocytes.

2. Discard the plasma supernatant and cells from Layer 1. Remove the polymorphonuclear leukocyte (PMN) layer (Layer 2) and place in a 17×100 mm polystyrene culture tube.

3. Wash the cells twice with 10 mL of PBS-BSA. Centrifuge at $300 \times$ g for 2 minutes each time. Decant the supernatant. Gently resuspend the cell button by manually rocking the tube. If the cell pellet appears pink (red blood cells present), proceed with lysing, step 4. If red blood cells are not visible, continue with step 5.

4. To lyse red blood cells, add 1 mL cold NH_4Cl solution to the resuspended granulocyte pellet. Incubate for 5 minutes on ice. Wash cells twice with 10 mL PBS-BSA, centrifuging at $300 \times$ g for 2 minutes each time. Repeat this step as necessary until red blood cells are no longer visible.

5. Add 2 mL 1% PFA to the resuspended granulocytes, and mix gently. Incubate for 5 minutes at 20°C to 24°C.

6. Wash cells 2 more times, as in step 3.

7. Gently resuspend the cells in 1 mL PBS-BSA.

8. Count the cells and adjust the concentration to 10 to 12×10^6/mL in PBS-BSA.

■ Test Procedure: Indirect Granulocyte Immunofluorescence

1. If frozen, thaw the antisera tubes 15 minutes before use. Remove the stoppers.

2. Thoroughly resuspend granulocytes using a transfer pipet and avoiding bubbles.

3. Add 40 μL of the granulocyte suspension to each tube using a micropipet. Gently mix cells and sera at low speed with a vortex mixer.

4. Incubate uncovered tubes at 37°C for 30 minutes in a dry-air incubator.

5. Fill a syringe with PBS-BSA. Add 1 mL PBS-BSA to each tube. Centrifuge at 1,000 × g for 1 minute. Decant the supernatant completely by vigorously flicking the tubes. Resuspend the cell button by manually flicking the tubes. Exert sufficient force to completely resuspend the cells, but not enough to damage the cell membranes. Repeat twice more.

6. To each tube, add 40 μL of the appropriate dilution of FITC-AHG using a micropipet. (We use FITC-AHG to total immunoglobulins for routine screening of sera.) Mix by gently rocking the tubes.

7. Incubate the tubes at 20°C to 24°C for 30 minutes in the dark.

8. Wash cells three times as in step 5.

9. Add 10 μL of glycerol-PBS to each tube using a micropipet. Gently tap the tubes on a flat surface to mix the glycerol-PBS with the cells.

10. Gently resuspend cells using a microliter syringe and disposable tip. Transfer 2 to 3 μL cell suspension to a clean printed microscope slide. Apply a coverglass and allow cells to settle in the dark for a minimum of 15 minutes before reading.

■ Test Procedure: Direct Granulocyte Immunofluorescence

1. If frozen, thaw the antisera tubes 15 minutes before use. Remove the stoppers.

2. Thoroughly resuspend granulocytes using a transfer pipet and avoiding bubbles.

3. Add 40 μL of the granulocyte suspension to each tube using a micropipet. Gently mix cells and sera at low speed with a vortex mixer.

4. Incubate uncovered tubes at 37°C for 30 minutes in a dry-air incubator.

5. Fill a syringe with PBS-BSA. Add 1 mL PBS-BSA to each tube. Centrifuge at 1,000 × g for 1 minute. Decant the supernatant completely by vigorously flicking the tubes. Resuspend the cell button by manually flicking the tubes. Exert sufficient force to completely resuspend the cells, but not enough to damage the cell membranes. Repeat once more.

6. Add 40 μL cell suspension to empty tubes for direct testing. Wash all cells one more time, as in step 5.

7. Add 40 µL of appropriate dilutions of FITC-AHG to each well (we use FITC-AHG to total immunoglobulins, IgG, IgM, and IgA for direct testing when sufficient granulocytes can be isolated). Mix by gently rocking the tray.

8. Incubate the tubes at 20°C to 24°C for 30 minutes in the dark.

9. Wash cells three times as in step 5.

10. Add 10 µL of glycerol-PBS to each tube using a micropipet. Gently tap the tubes on a flat surface to mix the glycerol-PBS with the cells.

11. Gently resuspend cells using a microliter syringe and disposable tip. Transfer 2 to 3 µL cell suspension to a clean printed microscope slide. Apply a coverglass and allow cells to settle in the dark for a minimum of 15 minutes before reading.

Interpretation of Results

Read the slides using a fluorescence microscope. The strengths of the reactions are graded 0 to 4, according to the characteristics of fluorescent staining.

Grade	Characteristic
0	No cell-bound fluorescence
±	Minimal cell-bound fluorescence
1	Fluorescent dots barely outline cell membrane distinctly
2	Fluorescence appears as closely-spaced but distinct dots on cell membrane
3	Fluorescent dots on cell membrane are partially merged to form bands
4	Fluorescence appears as solid ring around cell

Although minimized by the PFA-fixation of granulocytes and use of $F(ab')_2$ fragments of antihuman globulin, some nonspecific binding of immunoglobulins may still occur. Negative or 1+ reactions are acceptable for negative controls. Reactivity of negative controls must be used as the baseline for interpretation of other reactions with any panel cell.

Gentle handling is required to prevent damage to the granulocyte membranes. When damaged, cells will have cytoplasmic rather than membrane fluorescence and cannot be evaluated.

Positive reactions due to binding of immune complexes are not visually distinguishable from those caused by antibodies. Immune complexes may be excluded only when polymorphism is evident.

Normal donor cells may be tested in parallel with patients' cells to verify accurate dilutions of the conjugates in direct testing. They should demonstrate the appropriate reactions with positive and negative control sera, and direct testing of normal donor cells should be negative.

References

Lalezari P, Pryce SC: Detection of neutrophil and platelet antibodies in immunologically induced neutropenia and thrombocytopenia, in Rose NR, Friedmann H, (eds): *Manual of clinical immunology.* Washington, DC, American Society for Microbiology, pp 744–749, 1980.

Verheugt FWA, von dem Borne AEGKr, Decary S, et al: The detection of granulocyte alloantibodies with an indirect immunofluorescence test. *Brit J Haematol* 36:533–544, 1977.

2.5 Antibody-Dependent Lymphocyte-Mediated Granulocytotoxicity (ADLG)

Materials

1. Polystyrene culture tubes
   a. 16 × 150 mm
   b. 17 × 100 mm
2. 100 mL Nalgene beaker
3. 37°C incubator with 5% CO_2
4. Rotating platform mixer
5. Magnet
6. 17 × 120 mm polystyrene conical centrifuge tube (15 mL)
7. 30 mL syringe
8. 3.5 inch, 17 gauge spinal needle
9. Refrigerated centrifuge with horizontal rotor
10. 56°C incubator or water bath
11. Polystyrene U-bottom microtiter plate and sealers
12. 12 × 75 mm borosilicate culture tubes
13. Gamma counter

Reagents

1. Sodium heparin
2. Dextran
3. 0.9% saline solution
4. Carbonyl iron
5. Ficoll-Hypaque Solutions I & II (see procedure 1.1)
6. McCoy's 5a medium (Gibco)
   a. Without serum
   b. With 10% fetal calf serum

7. Sodium chloride (NaCl)

8. Potassium chloride (KCl)

9. Sodium phosphate, dibasic (Na_2HPO_4)

10. Potassium phosphate, monobasic (KH_2PO_4)

11. 10% disodium edetate (Na_2EDTA)

12. Sodium chromate (^{51}Cr): 1 mCi/mL

13. Sodium dodecyl sulfate (SDS)

Prepared Reagents

1. 5% dextran in 0.9% saline solution

2. Phosphate-buffered saline solution (PBS)

   a. Dissolve 8.0 g NaCl, 0.2 g KCl, 1.15 g Na_2HPO_4, and 0.2 g KH_2PO_4 in 1,000 mL distilled water.

   b. Adjust pH to 7.3.

3. Phosphate-buffered saline-EDTA solution (PBS-EDTA)

   a. Mix 500 mL PBS and 25 mL 10% Na_2EDTA.

   b. Adjust pH to 6.8.

4. 1% sodium dodecyl sulfate (SDS) in 0.9% saline solution

Method

NOTE: A diagrammatic summary of the method is shown in Figure 13–1 on the following page.

■ **Lymphocyte and Granulocyte Isolation**

1. Isolate granulocytes and lymphocytes from fresh whole blood anticoagulated with sodium heparin. Substitute 5% Dextran for 1% methyl cellulose in step 1 (see procedure 1.1). Process 100 to 160 mL of donor whole blood (depending upon absolute lymphocyte count) to obtain sufficient lymphocytes to test eight to ten specimens and/or controls.

2. Lymphocyte preparation

   a. Remove and discard the plasma supernatant from each conical tube until 3 to 4 mL remain above Layer 1. Remove the remaining plasma along with Layer 1. Pool the layers from all tubes in 100 mL Nalgene beaker.

   b. Place a large pea-sized amount of carbonyl iron into the beaker. Mix the cell suspension with the iron thoroughly, using a transfer pipet. Incubate the cell-iron suspension on a rotating platform with speed adjusted to provide thorough mixing without spilling (approximately 120 rpm) at 37°C for 20 minutes.

Figure 13–1.

Diagrammatic summary of the antibody-dependent lymphocyte-mediated granulocyte cytotoxicity (ADLG) assay.

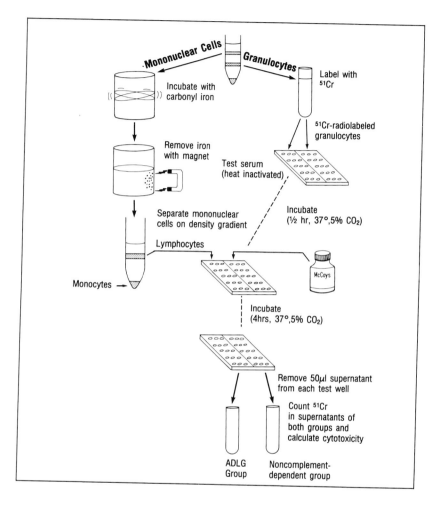

c. Remove the carbonyl iron using a magnet on the exterior of the beaker to bring iron down from sides into a lump at the bottom. Draw the lump of iron up the side of the beaker and discard it.

d. Place 5 mL aliquots of the lymphocyte suspension in 15 mL conical tubes. Wash the beaker with 5 mL 0.9% saline solution. Aliquot the saline solution among the tubes, not exceeding 6 mL of suspension in each tube. Mix the saline solution with the lymphocytes thoroughly.

e. Layer 3 mL of Solution I under the lymphocytes with the spinal needle and syringe. Centrifuge the tubes at 1,650 × g at 18°C for 15 minutes.

f. Aspirate and discard the plasma down to the lymphocyte layer. Remove the lymphocyte layer with the smallest amount of Ficoll-Hypaque possible, placing each layer into a separate 17 × 100 mm culture tube.

g. Fill each tube with McCoy's 5a medium without serum. Centrifuge at 800 × g for 8 to 10 minutes. Decant the supernatants, pool cell pellets, and wash again.

h. Decant the supernatant and add 1.0 mL of McCoy's 5a medium with 10% fetal bovine serum. Count the cells and adjust the concentration to 1.54×10^7 cells/mL.

3. Granulocyte preparation

a. Remove the granulocyte layers (Layer 2) of the original gradients. Place each layer in a separate 17 × 100 mm culture tube. Generally, four gradients yield adequate granulocytes for testing of 8 to 10 specimens and/or controls.

b. Fill each culture tube with PBS-EDTA. Centrifuge at 400 × g for 3 to 5 minutes. Decant the supernatant. Pool the cell pellets and wash again.

c. Decant the supernatant and resuspend the cells in 1 mL PBS-EDTA. Count and adjust the concentration to 1×10^7 cells/mL.

d. Transfer 1 mL of the cell suspension to a clean 17 × 100 mm culture tube. Add 200 μL ^{51}Cr. Mix well and incubate at 37°C for one hour. Gently mix cells by inversion every 10 minutes.

e. Add 4 mL PBS-EDTA to the culture tube with the labeled granulocytes. Centrifuge at 400 × g for 3 to 5 minutes. Decant the supernatant and resuspend the cells. Add PBS without EDTA. Centrifuge as before. Decant the supernatant and resuspend the cells.

f. Count the cells and adjust the concentration to 5×10^6 cells/mL in PBS without EDTA.

■ *Test Procedure*

1. Inactivate each serum by incubating at 56°C for 35 minutes. Mix thoroughly.

2. Pipet 10 μl of each serum or control into six consecutive wells of a microtiter tray. Each test or control serum is run in triplicate in both the noncomplement-dependent cytotoxicity and antibody-dependent lymphocyte-mediated granulocytotoxicity (ADLG) phases of the assay. Six wells of each of the following must also be included with each assay:

a. 1% SDS

b. AB serum

c. Two O-positive (negative control) sera

d. Two positive control sera

e. Patient or other sera to be studied

3. Add 10 μL of labeled granulocyte suspension to all wells. Place a sealer over the tray. Incubate in a 37°C incubator with 5% CO_2 for 30 minutes. Pipet 10 μL of the labeled granulocyte suspension into three 12 × 75 mm borosilicate tubes.

4. Add 130 μL 0.9% saline solution to each of the wells containing SDS. Add 130 μL McCoy's medium with 10% fetal bovine serum to three of the six wells of each group for the noncomplement-dependent cytotoxicity reaction. Add 130 μL lymphocyte suspension to the remaining three wells of each group for the ADLG reaction. Cover the tray, centrifuge at 100 × g for 2 minutes, and incubate at 37°C with 5% CO_2 for 4 hours.

5. Centrifuge at 170 × g for 10 minutes. Remove 50 μL of supernatant from each well, being careful not to touch the sides of the well or the cell button at the bottom, and place in a 12 × 75 mm borosilicate tube. Count all the tubes (including those from step 3) in a gamma counter for 1 minute each, using the appropriate settings for ^{51}Cr. Background is determined by averaging the counts of three empty 12 × 75 mm tubes.

■ **Calculations**

1. $\bar{x}$ SDS value = average of values of six wells containing 1% SDS (see test procedure 2a).

2. $\bar{x}$ spontaneous release = average of values of wells containing AB serum (see test procedure 2b).

   a. Three wells with added McCoy's 5a medium measuring non complement-dependent cytotoxicity

   b. Three wells with added lymphocytes measuring ADLG cytotoxicity

3. $\bar{x}$ serum value = average of values of wells containing serum or control (see test procedure 2).

   a. Three wells with added McCoy's 5a medium (noncomplement-dependent phase)

   b. Three wells with added lymphocytes (ADLG phase)

4. Calculate for each serum or control:

   a. Noncomplement-dependent cytotoxicity (%) =

   $$\frac{\bar{x} \text{ serum value (McCoy's)} - \bar{x} \text{ spontaneous (McCoy's)}}{\bar{x} \text{ SDS value} - \bar{x} \text{ spontaneous (McCoy's)}}$$
   × 100.

b. ADLG cytotoxicity (%) =

$$\frac{\bar{x} \text{ serum value (lymphocytes)} - \bar{x} \text{ spontaneous (lymphocytes)}}{\bar{x} \text{ SDS value} - \bar{x} \text{ spontaneous (lymphocytes)}}$$
$$\times 100.$$

5. 100% label value = average of values of three 12 × 75 mm tubes containing labeled granulocyte suspension (see test procedure 3).

6. Calculate for each run:

% spontaneous release =

$$3 \times \frac{\bar{x} \text{ spontaneous (lymphocytes)}}{\bar{x} \text{ 100% label value}} \times 100.$$

Interpretation of Results

Normal percent spontaneous release is 15% to 25%. Higher values may be due to granulocyte damage and/or poor labeling of granulocytes.

If the calculated percent of spontaneous release is greater than 30%, low levels of cytotoxicity may be masked by the spontaneous release of ^{51}Cr. In such cases the assay results are invalid.

The following criteria are used to determine positive reactions in our laboratory:

ABO-compatible tests > 4.8% cytotoxicity
ABO-incompatible tests > 10.0% cytotoxicity

ADLG cytotoxicity must also be at least 2.2 times the noncomplement-dependent cytotoxicity to be interpreted as a positive reaction. However, each laboratory performing ADLG should establish its own normal ranges.

References

Logue GL, Kurlander R, Pepe P, et al: Antibody-dependent lymphocyte-mediated granulocyte cytotoxicity in man. *Blood* 51:97–108, 1978.

Richards K, Sadrzadeh SMH, Clay M, et al: Antibody-dependent lymphocyte-mediated granulocytoxicity (ADLG) for the detection of granulocyte antibodies. *J Immunol Methods* 63:93–102, 1983.

2.6 Microlymphocytotoxicity Assay for Human Leukocyte Antigen (HLA) Antibody Detection

Materials

1. Repeating microliter dispenser and stream splitter

2. 72-well microtest tissue culture trays

3. Microliter syringes and repeating dispensers
   a. #1705 with disposable tips
   b. #725SN
4. −80°C freezer
5. Phase contrast microscope, inverted or standard with 10X objective

Reagents	1. Paraffin oil
	2. RPMI-1640 with Hepes buffer
	3. HLA-ABC Rabbit Complement (Pelfreez)
	4. 0.4% trypan blue
	5. Disodium edetate (Na_2EDTA)
	6. Barbitol buffer

Prepared Reagents	1. HLA-ABC Rabbit Complement: Titrate each new lot of complement with known positive and negative sera against known positive and negative lymphocyte donors. Select a dilution that demonstrates maximal specific activity with minimal nonspecific cytotoxicity.
	2. Trypan blue-EDTA solution
	a. Prepare 2% Na_2EDTA in barbitol buffer. Adjust pH to 7.0 to 7.4.
	b. Mix two parts 0.4% trypan blue with three parts EDTA barbitol buffer.

Method	■ *Selection and Preparation of Cell Panel*
	1. Isolate and prepare lymphocytes using the standard techniques described on pages 21–27 of *HLA Without Tears* (ASCP Press).
	2. Select 24 lymphocyte preparations so that all except extremely low frequency HLA-A, -B, and -C loci antigens are represented. Preparations may be either fresh or frozen and thawed immediately before use. All cell preparations must contain 90% to 100% viable lymphocytes free of granulocytes, red blood cells, and platelets.
	■ *Preparation of Antibody Screening Trays*
	1. Add 5 to 7 µL of paraffin oil to each well using a microliter dispenser and stream splitter. Use eight trays for each group of six sera to be screened.
	2. Add 1 µL of pooled human sera (PHS) under the oil in each well in all even-numbered rows using a microliter syringe and

disposable tip. This is a negative control and detects carryover due to high-titered antibodies.

3. Assign one serum to each odd numbered row. Add 1 μL of that serum to all six wells.

4. Store trays at −80°C until ready to use.

■ Test Procedure

1. Thaw antibody screening trays immediately before use.

2. Dilute selected lymphocyte preparations to a concentration of 2×10^6 cells/mL in RPMI-1640. Mix thoroughly.

3. Add 1 μL of each cell suspension to the serum in the appropriate wells. Test each cell-serum combination in duplicate, adding the first lymphocyte suspension to columns A and B, the second suspension to columns C and D, and the third suspension to columns E and F of the first tray. Continue, adding the remaining lymphocyte suspensions to the other trays.

4. Incubate at room temperature (20°C to 24°C) for 30 minutes.

5. Add 5 μL of diluted rabbit complement to each well, using a microliter syringe.

6. Incubate at room temperature for 60 minutes.

7. Remove excess complement by flicking or snapping trays with a quick motion of the wrist, being careful not to cast off the cells.

8. Fill each well with trypan blue-EDTA solution using a microliter dispenser and stream splitter, being careful not to disrupt the cells. Allow to stain for 10 minutes, then flick off excess dye as in step 7.

9. Add 5 μL of RPMI-1640 to each well with a microliter syringe to prevent evaporation. Allow cells to settle at least 10 minutes prior to reading.

Interpretation of Results

Read trays using a phase contrast microscope. Viable lymphocytes exclude dye and are small and refractile. Nonviable lymphocytes contain dye and are larger, flatter, and stained blue. Score reactions by estimating the percentage of cell death. Record results according to the following scale:

Score	Interpretation	% Nonviable Cells
1	Negative	0% to 15%
2	Weakly reactive	16% to 25%
4	Moderately reactive	26% to 50%
6	Positive	51% to 80%
8	Strongly positive	81% to 100%

References

Terasaki PI, Bernoco D, Park MS, et al: Microdroplet testing for HLA-A, -B, -C, and -D antigens. *Am J Clin Pathol* 69:103–120, 1978.

HLA Without Tears. Miller WV, Rodey G (eds). Chicago, American Society of Clinical Pathologists, 1981.

SECTION 3: Antibody Absorption and Elution

> ## 3.1 Absorption of Serum with Platelets for the Removal of Lymphocytotoxic Antibodies

Materials

1. 600 mL transfer pack units
2. Component centrifuge
3. Plasma extractor
4. Plasma transfer sets
5. 50 mL conical centrifuge tubes
6. 1 mL microcentrifuge tubes and stoppers
7. Tube rotator
8. Microcentrifuge
9. Refrigerated ultracentrifuge and tubes
10. Filter paper
11. Hemacytometer and microscope

Reagents

1. 50 to 100 units platelet concentrates (outdated within 1 month)
2. Sodium chloride (NaCl)
3. Potassium chloride (KCl)
4. Potassium phosphate, monobasic (KH_2PO_4)
5. Sodium phosphate, dibasic, hydrated ($Na_2HPO_4 \cdot 7H_2O$)
6. 0.2% thimerosal (Ethylmercurithiosalicylate)

Prepared Reagent

1. Phosphate-buffered saline solution (PBS)
   a. Dissolve 8.0 g NaCl, 0.2 g KCl, 0.2 g KH_2PO_4, and 2.17 g $Na_2HPO_4 \cdot 7H_2O$ in 1,000 mL distilled water.
   b. Adjust pH to 7.0.

   NOTE: A buffered saline solution from the assay in which the absorbed serum is to be tested may be used as an alternative solution.

Method

■ **Platelet Preparation**

1. Pool platelet concentrates in 600 mL transfer bags.

2. Centrifuge at 100 × g for 10 minutes to produce platelet-rich plasma (PRP).

3. Transfer the PRP to a new 600 mL transfer bag using a plasma extractor, leaving behind any sedimented red blood cells.

4. Centrifuge the PRP at 2,500 × g for 10 minutes.

5. Drain the supernatant plasma off of the platelet pellet using transfer tubing and a plasma extractor and discard.

6. Transfer the platelets to 50 mL conical tubes, filling each tube with 15 to 20 mL of platelet suspension. Rinse any remaining platelets from the transfer bag with PBS and add to the tubes.

7. Fill tubes with PBS, mix, and centrifuge at 2,500 × g for 10 minutes.

8. Decant the supernatant. Transfer the platelet pellets to clean conical tubes, leaving any red blood cells in the original tubes.

9. Fill the conical tubes containing platelets with PBS. Mix and centrifuge at 100 × g for 5 minutes.

10. Transfer the PRP to clean 50 mL conical tubes and discard the pellets.

11. Centrifuge the PRP at 2,500 × g for 10 minutes.

12. Discard the supernatant plasma and transfer the platelet pellet to a clean tube, leaving behind the red blood cells.

13. Resuspend the platelet pellet in an equal volume of PBS.

14. Prepare a 1:100 dilution of the platelet suspension in PBS and examine on a hemacytometer to verify the purity of the platelet suspension. Fewer than 10 white blood cells per mm² should be present. If larger numbers of contaminating cells are present, repeat steps 9 through 12 above until the desired purity is attained.

15. Add 0.2 mL of 0.2% thimerosal for each 10 mL of platelet suspension. Store at 4°C to 6°C for up to 1 month. Discard if a rancid odor is present.

NOTE: Sometimes it is desirable to remove human leukocyte antigen (HLA) antibodies directed against a specific donor, such as the father in cases of alloimmune neonatal neutropenia (ANN), or a blood donor or recipient involved in a transfusion reaction. In such situations, absorption of the serum with cells of the specific donor is more effective. The mononuclear layer (Layer 1) of a discontinuous double-density gradient containing platelets and lymphocytes but virtually free of granulocytes (see procedure 1.1) may be washed and used for absorptions.

■ Absorption of Serum

1. For each 0.5 mL of serum to be absorbed, fill two 1mL microcentrifuge tubes with platelet suspension. Centrifuge for 5 minutes at 6,000 × g. Aspirate the supernatant and discard.

2. Resuspend the platelet pellet in PBS. Centrifuge at $6,000 \times$ g for 5 minutes. Aspirate the supernatant and discard. Repeat once more.

3. Centrifuge the platelet pellet at $6,000 \times$ g for 5 minutes. Blot the packed platelets with filter paper to avoid diluting serum with excess PBS. The platelet volume should be approximately 0.5 mL.

4. Fill half of the microcentrifuge tubes containing washed platelets with an equal volume of the serum to be absorbed. (The ratio of serum to platelets should be approximately 1:1 to 1.5:1.) A larger ratio of platelets to serum may be used for absorption when a strong lymphocytotoxic antibody is present (eg, 2 or 3 volumes of platelets to 1 volume of serum). One or two additional absorptions with fresh platelets may also be performed as an alternate technique.

5. Resuspend the platelets in the serum, stopper the tubes and rotate at 20°C to 24°C for 60 minutes.

6. Centrifuge the serum and platelets at $6,000 \times$ g for 5 minutes.

7. Transfer the serum to a tube with fresh washed, packed platelets and repeat steps 5 and 6 above.

8. Transfer the serum to ultracentrifuge tubes. Centrifuge at $13,000 \times$ g for 10 minutes to remove platelet debris.

9. Transfer the serum to a clean tube without disturbing sedimented pellet. Store at -80°C until tested.

10. Verify the removal of HLA antibodies by testing the absorbed serum in the lymphocytotoxicity assay.

3.2 Absorption Methods for Determination of Antigen Cell Line Distribution

3.2–A   Granulocytes

Materials
1. Microcentrifuge and tubes
2. Dry-air incubator or water bath

Cell Preparation
Isolate purified granulocytes using gradients of Ficoll-Hypaque or Percoll (see procedures 1.1, 1.2).

Absorption	1.	Incubate 0.1 mL serum with 10^7 granulocytes at 37°C for 1 hour, with rotation or occasional mixing.
	2.	Centrifuge at 6,000 × g for 5 minutes to remove cell debris.

3.2–B   Red Blood Cells

Materials	1.	Microcentrifuge and tubes
	2.	Dry-air incubator or water bath
	3.	Hemacytometer and microscope

Reagent	1.	0.9% saline solution

Cell Preparation	1.	Pool anticoagulated whole blood from two to four type O donors.
	2.	Wash red blood cells with 0.9% saline solution three times, each time centrifuging at 100 × g for 10 minutes and discarding the supernatant.
	3.	Microscopically verify the removal of leukocytes and platelets.

Absorption	1.	Incubate serum with an equal volume of washed, packed red blood cells at 37°C for 1 hour.
	2.	Centrifuge at 6,000 × g for 5 minutes to remove cell debris.

3.2–C   Platelets

1. Perform platelet preparation and absorption as described previously (see procedure 3.1).

3.2–D   Monocytes

Materials	1.	17 × 120 mm conical centrifuge tubes (15 mL)
	2.	17 × 100 mm polystyrene culture tubes
	3.	Refrigerated centrifuge with horizontal rotor
	4.	Plastic Petri dishes
	5.	37°C incubator with 5% CO_2

6. Siliconized rubber spatula

7. Microscope and slide

Reagents

1. Phosphate-buffered saline solution (PBS). Adjust pH to 7.2.

2. Ficoll-Hypaque Solution I (see procedure 1.1)

3. RPMI-1640 (Gibco)

4. RPMI-1640 with 5% human serum

5. Hank's balanced salt solution (HBSS) (Gibco)

6. 10 mM EDTA in phosphate-buffered saline solution

7. Wright's stain

Cell Preparation

1. Place 7 mL aliquots of a discarded, buffy-coat fraction (approximately 100 mL) from the preparation of a leukocyte-poor plateletpheresis product in conical tubes.

2. Add 7 mL PBS to each tube. Centrifuge at 1,650 × g for 5 minutes. Remove the buffy-coat layers.

3. Layer 7 mL aliquots of washed buffy coats over 7 mL of Ficoll-Hypaque Solution I in conical centrifuge tubes. Centrifuge at 1,650 × g at 18°C for 15 minutes.

4. Discard the plasma. Transfer cells at the plasma-Ficoll-Hypaque interface to 17 × 100 mm culture tubes. Add RPMI-1640 with 5% normal human serum. Centrifuge at 300 × g for 5 minutes. Discard the supernatant.

5. Resuspend the cells in RPMI with 5% human serum to a concentration of 5×10^7/mL.

6. Layer onto plastic Petri dishes (approximately 1.5 mL/dish). Incubate at 37°C in 5% CO_2 in air for 90 minutes.

7. To remove nonadherent cells, wash five times with warm HBSS, vigorously swirling plates. Between washes, decant wash solution completely.

8. Add 1 to 2 mL 10 mM EDTA in PBS to each plate. Scrape plate with a siliconized rubber spatula. Decant and save the solution with cells. Repeat and pool cells.

9. Centrifuge the cell suspension at 600 × g for 10 minutes. Mix a drop of cell suspension with a few drops of human serum. Spread on a microscope slide. Allow to dry. Stain with Wright's stain and examine microscopically.

10. The cell suspension should contain approximately 75% to 90% monocytes. The other cells should be predominantly lymphocytes with no neutrophils.

Absorption	*1.*	Incubate 0.1 mL serum with 10^7 cells at 37°C for 60 minutes.
	2.	Centrifuge at 6,000 × g for 5 minutes to remove cell debris.

3.2–E   Lymphocytes

Materials	*1.*	Microcentrifuge and tubes
	2.	Dry-air incubator or water bath

Cell Preparation	*1.*	Isolate T- and B-lymphocytes using the standard nylon adherence techniques described in sections 1-8-1 to 1-8-6 of *Nylon Wool Separation of T and B Lymphocytes* (The American Association for Clinical Histocompatibility Testing).

Absorption	*1.*	Incubate 0.1 mL serum with 10^7 T-lymphocytes and another aliquot of 0.1 mL serum with 10^7 B-lymphocytes, each at 37°C for 1 hour.
	2.	Centrifuge at 6,000 × g for 5 minutes to remove cell debris.

Interpretation of Results (Sections 3.2–A to 3.2–E)	Due to varying strengths of antibodies and/or the number of antigen sites on various cell lines, absorptions performed under these conditions may be incomplete. Therefore, it is suggested that unabsorbed and absorbed sera be titrated and tested in parallel. A significant decrease in titer (4-fold or greater) of the absorbed serum may indicate presence of antigen on the absorbing cell membrane, even though some reactivity remains. Use repeated absorption(s) of diluted serum to confirm this.

References	Lopez-Bernstein G, Reuben J, Hersh E, et al: Comparative functional analysis of lymphocytes and monocytes from plateletpheresis. *Transfusion* 23:201–206, 1983.
	Fotino M, Menon AK: *Nylon Wool Separation of T and B Lymphocytes*, in Zachery A, Braun W (eds). New York, the American Association for Clinical Histocompatibility Testing, 1-8-1 to 1-8-6, 1981.

3.3 Elution of Granulocyte Antibodies

COMMENT: Method 3.3 is not regularly performed in our lab but is included for completeness of available methods. We have encountered problems performing this method. The source of this previously published method is: von dem Borne AEGKr, van der Plas-van Dalen C, Engelfriet CP: Immunofluorescence antiglobulin test, in McMillan R (ed): *Immune cytopenias*. New York, Churchill Livingston, pp 106–127, 1983.

Materials	1. 50 mL conical centrifuge tube
	2. Centrifuge
	3. Ultrafilters with 95 mm diameter membranes (Amicon) and nitrogen pressure apparatus
	4. Magnetic stirrer
	5. Dialysis tubing

Reagents	1. Bovine serum albumin (BSA)
	2. Phosphate-buffered saline solution (PBS)
	3. Disodium edetate (Na_2EDTA)
	4. Sodium chloride (NaCl)
	5. Trisodium citrate ($C_6H_5Na_3O_7$)
	6. Citric acid ($C_6H_8O_7$)
	7. Sodium hydroxide (NaOH)

Prepared Reagents	1. 0.2% bovine serum albumin in phosphate-buffered saline (PBS-BSA):
	2. PBS-EDTA: 2% (w/v) Na_2EDTA in PBS
	3. Elution buffer: 0.1 M trisodium citrate in 1.0 M NaCl added to a solution of 1.0 M citric acid in 1.0 M NaCl until pH reaches 2.8
	4. Neutralizing solution: 0.04 M NaOH in 0.14 M NaCl

Method	1. Suspend sensitized granulocytes in 0.5 mL PBS-BSA to a concentration of 5 to 10×10^6.
	CAUTION: False negative results may occur when too few granulocytes are used for eluate preparation.
	2. Stirring constantly, add elution buffer by drops to the granulocyte suspension, until pH reaches 2.8.
	3. Incubate at room temperature for 10 minutes.
	4. Centrifuge at $200 \times g$ for 5 minutes. Transfer the supernatant to a 50 mL centrifuge tube. Add neutralizing solution immediately until pH reaches 7.2.

5. Concentrate the eluate to an approximate volume of 0.5 mL using a 95 mm diameter ultrafilter under a pressure of 3 kg/cm^2 (nitrogen) with continuous magnetic stirring.

6. Dialyze the concentrated eluate against PBS-EDTA.

7. Test eluates by granulocyte immunofluorescence or agglutination.

Reference   Helmerhorst FM, van Oss CJ, Bruynes ECE, et al: Elution of granulocyte and platelet antibodies. *Vox Sang* 43:196–204, 1982.

SECTION 4: Isolation of Serum Immunoglobulin Fractions

4.1 Isolation of IgG Fraction

Materials
1. 0.2 μm filter
2. Chromatography column with support system
3. Dialysis tubing
4. Fraction collector and tubes
5. Spectrophotometer

Reagents
1. Potassium phosphate, dibasic (K_2HPO_4)
2. Sodium azide (NaN_3)
3. DEAE-Affi-Gel Blue (Bio-Rad Laboratories)

Prepared Reagent
1. Buffer: 0.02M K_2HPO_4 with 0.2% sodium azide. Adjust pH to 8.0.

Method
1. Pass serum through a 0.2 μm filter to remove aggregated protein.
2. Dialyze the serum sample against three changes of buffer at 4°C over a period of 2 to 3 days.
3. Prepare a column of DEAE-Affi-Gel Blue with a total bed volume of 7 mL per mL of serum to be fractionated as instructed by manufacturer.
4. Prewash the column with 2 bed volumes of buffer. Apply the serum sample to the column.
5. Elute the IgG fraction with 3 volumes of buffer. Collect fractions, pooling the protein peak (determined by measuring absorbance at 280 nm).
6. Quantitate the protein by the method of Lowry or Bradford. Concentrate to the desired protein concentration.

References

DEAE-Affi-Gel Blue purifies IgG (product bulletin #1062). Richmond, CA, Bio-Rad Laboratories, 1982.

Bio-Rad protein assay (product bulletin #1069). Richmond, CA, Bio-Rad Laboratories, 1982.

Harkee EF: Determination of protein: A modification of the Lowry method that gives a linear photometric response. *Anal Biochem* 48:422–427, 1972.

Bradford MM: A rapid and sensitive method for the quantitation of microgram quantities of protein utilizing the principle of protein-dye binding. *Anal Biochem* 72:248–254, 1976.

4.2 Isolation of IgM Fraction

Materials
1. 0.2 μm filter
2. 15 × 90 cm chromatography column and support system
3. Fraction collector and tubes
4. Spectrophotometer

Reagents
1. Tromethamine (TRIS)
2. Sodium chloride (NaCl)
3. Sodium azide (NaN$_3$)
4. Hydrochloric acid (HCl)
5. Sephacryl S-300 Superfine (Pharmacia), MW range = 10,000 to 1.5×10^6

Prepared Reagent
1. 0.1 M TRIS in 0.5M NaCl buffer with 0.02% sodium azide. Adjust pH to 8.0 with HCl.

Method
1. Pass serum through a 0.2 μm filter to remove aggregated protein.
2. Prepare a 15 × 90 cm column with Sephacryl S-300.
3. Prewash the column with 2 bed volumes of TRIS buffer at 0.9 mL/minute. Apply the serum sample to the column.
4. Collect 3 mL fractions at 0.5 mL/minute. Determine the protein content using uv absorbance at 280 nm.
5. Test all fractions, from the void volume to the midpoint of the first major peak (IgG) for IgG and IgM (see procedure 4.3).
6. Pool fractions containing only IgM. Concentrate if necessary.

Reference
Gel filtration theory and practice (pamphlet). Piscataway, NJ, Pharmacia Fine Chemicals, 1985.

4.3-A Ouchterlony Double Agar Diffusion

Materials	*1.* Water bath or stirring hot plate
	2. 3 × 1 inch glass slides
	3. 1 mm punch
	4. Petri dishes

Reagents	*1.* Agar (Difco)
	2. Glycine
	3. Sodium chloride (NaCl)
	4. 1 N sodium hydroxide (NaOH)
	5. Disodium edetate (Na_2EDTA)
	6. Sodium azide (NaN_3)
	7. 10% sodium carbonate (Na_2CO_3).
	8. Rabbit anti-human antisera (IgG, IgM, albumin, transferrin, whole serum)

Prepared Reagents	*1.* EDTA-glycine-saline buffer
	a. Dissolve 7.5 g glycine, 8.5 g NaCl, 5.0 mL 1 N NaOH, and 3.75 g Na_2EDTA in 750 mL distilled water.
	b. Adjust pH to 8.2 with 10% Na_2CO_3.
	c. Add water to bring volume to 1,000 mL.
	d. Add sodium azide to bring the final concentration to 0.02%.
	2. 1% agar in EDTA-glycine-saline buffer: Boil until dissolved.

Method	*1.* Melt the 1% agar using a boiling water bath or stirring hot plate.
	2. Dispense 3 mL 1% agar onto 3 × 1 inch glass slides on a level surface. Cool.
	3. Punch wells 1 mm in diameter in the desired pattern. Fill outer wells with column fractions. Fill center wells with antisera.
	4. Place the slides on a damp paper towel and cover with Petri dishes. Incubate overnight at room temperature (20°C to 24°C).

5. Read and record precipitation patterns.

Reference   Johnson AM. Immunoprecipitation in gels, in Rose NR, Friedman H, Fahey JL (eds): *Manual of Clinical Laboratory Immunology.* Washington, DC, American Society for Microbiology, pp 14–24, 1986.

4.3–B   Immunoelectrophoresis (IEP)

Materials
1. Water bath or stirring hot plate
2. 3×1 inch glass slides
3. Electrophoresis apparatus
4. Whatman #1 filter paper
5. Petri dishes

Reagents
1. Agar (Difco)
2. Sodium barbital
3. Sodium acetate $\cdot 3H_2O$
4. Disodium edetate (Na_2EDTA)
5. 4 N sodium hydroxide (NaOH)
6. Sodium azide (NaN_3)
7. Bromphenol blue tracking dye
8. Rabbit anti-human antisera

Prepared Reagents
1. Barbital buffer
   a. Dissolve 9.75 g sodium barbital, 6.50 g sodium acetate $\cdot 3H_2O$, and 3.72 g Na_2EDTA in 900 mL distilled water.
   b. Adjust pH to 8.6 using 4 N NaOH. Bring volume to 1,000 mL.
   c. Add sodium azide to bring the final concentration to 0.02%.
2. 1.5% agar in barbital buffer: Boil until dissolved.

Method
1. Melt the 1.5% agar in a boiling water bath or stirring hot plate.
2. Dispense 3 mL 1.5% agar onto 3×1 inch glass slides on a level surface. Cool.
3. Cut wells and troughs as needed for samples.
4. Remove the wells and fill with samples, leaving troughs in place. Place bromphenol blue tracking dye in one well.

5. Assemble electropheresis apparatus, filling buffer reservoirs with barbital buffer and using Whatman #1 filter paper wicks.

6. Run at 120 volts (constant voltage) for 2 hours or until tracking dye is near the end of the trough.

7. Remove troughs from slides and fill with antisera.

8. Place slides on a damp paper towel and cover with Petri dishes. Incubate overnight at room temperature (20°C to 24°C).

9. Read and record precipitation lines to identify components.

Reference Mehl VS, Penn GM. Electrophoretic and immunochemical characterization of immunoglobulins, in Rose NR, Friedman H, Fahey JL, (eds): *Manual of Clinical Laboratory Immunology*. Washington, DC, American Society for Microbiology, pp 126–137, 1986.

4.4 Concentration of Column Fractions

Materials
1. Dialysis tubing
2. Centrifuge
3. Centriflo membrane cones (Amicon)

Reagent
1. Phosphate-buffered saline solution (PBS). Adjust pH to 7.2

Method
1. Dialyze pooled fractions containing the desired component against PBS.

2. Test the fractions and the unfractionated serum for the desired component with Mancini radial immunodiffusion or other suitable method. This permits calculation of the dilution factor of the serum fraction relative to the starting material.

3. Concentrate pooled fractions by centrifuging at $1,000 \times g$ in Centriflo membrane cones according to the manufacturer's instructions until the desired concentration is obtained.

SECTION 5: Miscellaneous Procedures

5.1 Chloroquine Stripping of Human Leukocyte Antigens (HLA)

COMMENT: Method 5.1 is not regularly performed in our lab but is included for completeness of available methods. We have encountered problems performing this method. The source of this previously published method is: Minchinton RM, Waters AH: Chloroquine stripping of HLA antigens from neutrophils without removal of neutrophil-specific antigens. *Brit J Haematol* 57:703–706, 1984.

Reagents

1. Chloroquine disphosphate salt

2. Phosphate-buffered saline solution (PBS)

3. Bovine serum albumin (BSA)

Prepared Reagents

1. Chloroquine solution: 200 mg/mL chloroquine diphosphate salt in PBS. Adjust pH to 5.0.

2. 0.2% bovine serum albumin in PBS (PBS-BSA)

Method

1. Suspend isolated granulocytes in 5 to 7 mL fresh chloroquine solution.

2. Incubate in darkness for 2 hours at room temperature; mix occasionally.

3. Wash treated cells three times in PBS-BSA.

4. Fix cells before testing in granulocyte immunofluorescence.

NOTE: This method is reported to remove HLA but not neutrophil-specific antigens from granulocytes when tested in the granulocyte immunofluorescence assay. However, we have experienced difficulties with this method due to 1) damage to cell membranes, 2) cell clumping, 3) inconsistent removal of HLA antigens, and 4) occasional loss of neutrophil-specific antigens. The source of chloroquine may be critical to this procedure.

5.2 Recalcification of Reagent Plasma

Materials
1. 1,000 mL glass beaker
2. Magnetic stirring device and stir bar
3. 50 mL polypropylene conical tubes
4. Centrifuge
5. Micropore filters
   - a. 1.2 μm
   - b. 0.45 μm

Reagents
1. Calcium chloride dihydrate ($CaCl_2 \cdot 2H_2O$)
2. Topical human thrombin

Prepared Reagent
1. 1 M Calcium chloride: Dissolve 14.7 g $CaCl_2 \cdot 2H_2O$ in 100 mL distilled water. Prepare fresh on the day of use.

Method
1. Place the plasma in a 1,000 mL glass beaker.
2. Add 2 mL of 1M calcium chloride for each 100 mL of plasma in the beaker.
3. Add a stir bar to the plasma and place the beaker on a magnetic stirring device. Set the control at a speed which minimizes foaming of the plasma.
4. Stir the plasma at room temperature (20°C to 24°C) until a clot forms around the stir bar, about 2 to 3 hours. If formation of a clot is minimal or inadequate, add 0.5 mL thrombin for each 250 mL plasma to enhance clotting. Addition of more thrombin may be necessary if clot formation does not begin within 1 hour.
5. Incubate the plasma along with the clot overnight at 4°C to 6°C to allow clot retraction.
6. Decant the recalcified plasma off the clot into a clean container. Manually squeeze any remaining plasma from the clot and discard the clot.
7. Transfer the plasma to 50 mL conical tubes. Centrifuge at 3,400 $\times$ g for 30 minutes.
8. Filter the supernatant plasma with a 1.2 μm filter, followed by a 0.45 μm filter.
9. Transfer the filtered plasma to suitable containers for storage.

SECTION 6: Indium 111 In Vivo Studies

6.1 Indium 111 Granulocyte Kinetic Studies

Materials

1. 16 × 150 mm culture tubes, sterile
2. 17 × 120 mm conical centrifuge tubes (15 mL), sterile
3. Laminar flow hood
4. Refrigerated centrifuge with horizontal rotor
5. 17 × 100 mm polystyrene tubes, sterile
6. Pasteur pipets, sterile
7. Syringes, sterile
   a. 3 mL
   b. 6 mL
8. Filter needles (Monoject)
9. 12 × 75 mm polystyrene tubes
10. 10 μL pipets
11. White blood cell (WBC) diluting pipets
12. Pipet shakers
13. Microscope
14. Gamma counter
15. Evacuated tubes
    a. 7 mL disodium edetate (Na_2EDTA)
    b. 10 mL serum
16. Hematocrit tubes
17. Micro-hematocrit centrifuge
18. 12 × 75 mm borosilicate counting tubes
19. Semilog graph paper

Reagents

1. Acid citrate dextrose (ACD), formula A
2. 6% hetastarch in 0.9% saline solution (American Critical Care)
3. 0.9% saline solution, sterile for injection
4. 25% normal human serum albumin (Cutter)
5. Indium 111–oxine, 1 mCi (Amersham)

| **Prepared Reagent** | *1.* 0.5% human serum albumin in sterile 0.9% saline solution |

| **Method** | ■ **Preparation and Labeling of Granulocytes** |

Method for Indium 111 Granulocyte Kinetic Studies

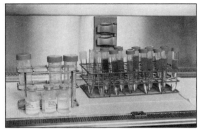

13–2 Granulocytes are isolated using sterile technique under a laminar flow hood.

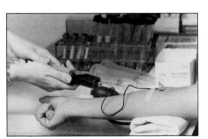

13–3 Whole blood for granulocyte isolation is obtained from the donor.

CAUTION: Except during centrifugation, perform procedures under a laminar flow hood using *sterile* technique, transfer equipment, and solutions (Figure 13–2).

Notes _____

_____

_____

_____

_____

_____

1. Collect 150 to 180 mL venous blood (or 30 mL of a leukapheresis product) (Figure 13–3). Dispense into sterile 16 × 150 mm tubes containing ACD anticoagulant (1.7 mL ACD per 10 mL blood).

Notes _____

_____

_____

_____

2. Add 3 mL hetastarch to each tube. Mix gently and position in a rack at approximately 30° angle for 20 to 30 minutes to sediment the red blood cells. (For leukapheresis cells, no additional hetastarch is added as it is used during the collection procedure.)

3. Remove the leukocyte-rich plasma and layer in 9 mL aliquots onto Ficoll-Hypaque double density gradients (see procedure 1.1).

CAUTION: Gradients must be found nonpyrogenic by an approved method and be sterile.

4. Centrifuge the gradient tubes at 1,650 × g at 18°C for 15 minutes.

5. Discard the supernatant portions and transfer each granulocyte layer (Layer 2) to a sterile 17 × 100 mm polystyrene tube using a sterile pipet.

6. Wash twice with 10 mL of 0.5% human serum albumin, centrifuging at 400 × g at 18°C for 5 minutes.

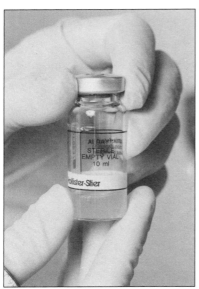

13-4 Isolated granulocytes are added to indium 111-oxine in a sterile vial, which is then placed behind a lead shield during incubation.

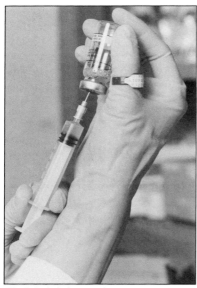

13-5 Labeled granulocytes are withdrawn from the vial through a filter needle, which is then discarded before infusion of cells into the recipient.

7. Combine and resuspend the washed granulocytes in 5 mL of sterile saline solution without albumin.

8. With a sterile pipet, gently transfer the granulocyte suspension to a sterile vial containing the indium 111–oxine (Figure 13–4).

Notes _____

9. Mix by gentle inversion and keep at room temperature for 30 minutes with gentle mixing about every 10 minutes.

10. Thoroughly resuspend the labeled granulocytes and withdraw them from the vial through a filter needle (Figure 13–5). Save the vial for later use.

Notes _____

11. Remove the filter needle and dispense 2 to 3 drops of cell suspension into a 12 × 75 mm polystyrene tube. From this sample:

    a. Dispense 10 μL of cell suspension into each of four 12 × 75 mm borosilicate counting tubes containing 1 mL of saline solution.

    b. Do a white blood cell count; the desired total number of granulocytes is 2 to 4 × 10^8 (minimum is 1 × 10^8).

    c. Do a red blood cell count if there are any visible red blood cells. Assume less than 10% if none are visible. For good kinetic data, red blood cells should be less than 10%. If greater than 20%, a decision would have to be made whether to inject. Results would be influenced by labeled red blood cells.

    d. Fill two capillary hematocrit tubes with the cell suspension. Centrifuge for 4 minutes. Break the tubes within 1 mm of the cell supernatant interface. Place the cell portions in 1 counting tube and the supernatant portions in another. These are the pre-injection cells and supernatant samples.

12. Replace the filter needle with a regular needle or butterfly infusion set. Record the volume to be injected and the recipient's height, weight, and sex.

■ Injection of Labeled Granulocytes

1. Infuse the cells directly into the recipient's vein, rinsing the butterfly tubing and/or syringe with the recipient's blood or 6 to 10 mL sterile saline solution.

    NOTE: If venous access is limited, the granulocytes can be injected through an existing intravenous line. Select an injection position as close as possible to the vein. Rinse the line with sterile saline solution, inject the labeled cells, and rinse with additional sterile saline solution. Do not inject the labeled cells directly into the lines containing anything other than normal saline solution.

2. Fill two capillary tubes from the small amount of cell suspension remaining in the labeling vial. Centrifuge for 4 minutes. Break the capillary tubes within 1 mm of the cell supernatant. Place the cell portion in one counting vial and the supernatant portion in another. These are the post-injection cells and supernatant samples.

■ Post-Injection Blood Samples

Following injection, 7 mL blood samples in EDTA should be obtained at 10 minutes, 30 minutes, 1 hour, 2 hours, 3 hours, 4 hours, 5 hours, and 6 hours if the recipient is equipped with a heparin lock. For patient studies in which the number of blood samples is restricted, samples should be drawn at 10 minutes, 1 hour, 2 hours, 4 hours, and 6 hours. The post-injection blood samples cannot be drawn through the same line used for injection of labeled cells. Each sample must be processed as follows:

1. Mix sample thoroughly.

2. Determine the hematocrit and white blood cell count (on the initial blood sample only).

3. Put 2 mL of whole blood in one counting tube and 1 mL of whole blood in another.

4. Centrifuge the remaining whole blood at $600 \times g$ for 5 minutes. Transfer the plasma to a 12×75 mm polystyrene tube and centrifuge at $600 \times g$ for 5 minutes. Check visually for the presence of cells. Put 1 mL of cell-free plasma in a counting tube.

5. Count samples for 1 minute on correct settings for indium 111 in a gamma counter. Determine background by counting 1 mL saline.

■ **Calculations**

1. Total radioactivity injected (total cpm)

    a. Average the counts for the quadruplicate 10 μL samples of the labeled granulocyte suspension (see preparation and labeling procedure 11a). The mean $= \dfrac{\text{cpm}}{10\ \mu\text{L}}$.

    b. Total cpm injected $= \dfrac{\text{cpm}}{10\ \mu\text{L}} \times$ total volume injected (μL).

       For example, if counts on 10 μL samples average 1,000,000 cpm and the volume injected is 5.0 mL, then total cpm injected $=$

$$\frac{1,000,000}{10} \times 5,000 = 500,000,000.$$

2. Obtain the blood volume of the recipient from the Tulane Tables based on height, weight, and sex.

3. Total radioactivity injected per mL of recipient's blood (cpm/mL)

    Radioactivity per mL of recipient's blood $=$

$$\frac{\text{total radioactivity injected (cpm) (see calculation 1)}}{\text{total blood volume (see calculation 2)}}.$$

    Using this example, $\dfrac{500,000,000}{5,800} = 86,207\ \dfrac{\text{cpm}}{\text{mL}}$.

This is the expected value obtained if all of the injected radioactivity remained in the circulation of the recipient.

4. Percentage of cell-associated radioactivity

a. Determine the mean cpm for the pre-injection cells and pre-injection supernatant samples (see preparation and labeling procedure 11d).

b. Determine the mean cpm for the post-injection cells and post-injection supernatant.

c. Pre-injection percent cell-associated radioactivity =

$$\frac{\text{pre-injection cells (cpm)}}{\text{pre-injection cells (cpm)} + \text{pre-injection supernatant (cpm)}} \times 100.$$

Post-injection percent cell-associated radioactivity =

$$\frac{\text{post-injection cells (cpm)}}{\text{post-injection cells (cpm)} + \text{post-injection supernatant (cpm)}} \times 100.$$

Both the pre-injection and post-injection samples are calculated because there may be a long delay between labeling and injection of the cells. Additional labeling of the cells can occur during this time, making the post-injection percent of cell-associated radioactivity higher. If the pre-injection and post-injection values are within 5% to 10% of each other, use the mean for further calculations. If the post-injection percentage is considerably higher, it should be used.

CAUTION: If the cells are not resuspended well at the time they are removed into the syringe for injection, the post-injection cpm may be higher because of a higher concentration of cells. Verify that the total cpm per capillary (ie, cells and supernatant) for pre-injection and post-injection samples are similar.

For example:

pre-injection cells = 130,000
pre-injection supernatant = 20,000 cpm

pre-injection percent cell-associated radioactivity =

$$\frac{130,000}{130,000 + 20,000} \times 100 = 86.7\%.$$

post-injection cells = 137,000 cpm
post-injection supernatant = 16,000 cpm

post-injection percent cell-associated radioactivity =

$$\frac{137,000}{137,000 + 16,000} \times 100 = 89.5\%.$$

Average of 86.7 + 89.5 = 88.1% cell-associated radioactivity.

5. Expected cell-associated radioactivity per mL of recipient's blood

    a. If all of the labeled cells remain in circulation (100% recovery) then the expected cell-associated radioactivity per mL = the injected radioactivity per mL (see calculation 3) × the percent cell-associated radioactivity (see calculation 4).

        For example, expected cell-associated radioactivity per mL =

$$86{,}207 \ \frac{\text{cpm}}{\text{mL}} \times 0.881 = 75{,}948 \ \text{cpm/mL}.$$

6. Intravascular recovery or percent of injected cell-associated radioactivity remaining in circulation

    Calculate the following for each post-injection blood sample:

    a. cpm per mL recipient's whole blood: Add the cpm value from the 2 mL and 1 mL whole blood samples (see post-injection blood sample procedure 3). Divide by 3.

        For example, if the cpm on 2 mL whole blood is 48,800 and the cpm on 1 mL whole blood is 25,900, then the average cpm per mL of recipient whole blood =

$$\frac{48{,}800 \ + \ 25{,}900}{3} = 24{,}900.$$

    This value includes both the cell-associated radioactivity and the plasma radioactivity.

    b. Plasma radioactivity (cpm) per mL whole blood: Multiply the cpm value for 1 mL plasma (see post-injection blood sample procedure 4) by 1 − hematocrit (see post-injection blood sample procedure 2).

        For example, if the cpm/mL plasma is 1,500 cpm and recipient's hematocrit is 42%, then the plasma cpm/mL whole blood =

$$1{,}500 \times (1 \ - \ .42) = 1{,}500 \times .58 = 870.$$

    This count represents the contribution of plasma radioactivity to the whole blood radioactivity.

    c. Actual cell-associated radioactivity per mL whole blood: cpm/mL whole blood (see calculation 6a)—plasma cpm/mL whole blood (see calculation 6b).

        For example: 24,900 − 870 = 24,030.

    d. Intravascular percent recovery: The intravascular percent recovery at the time the blood sample was drawn is equal to the *actual* cell-associated radioactivity per mL of recipient whole blood (see calculation 6c) divided by the expected cell-associated radioactivity per mL (see calculation 5).

For example, if the actual cell-associated radioactivity per mL is 24,030 (see calculation 6c) and the expected cell-associated per mL is 75,948 (see calculation 5):

$$\text{The intravascular recovery} = \frac{24,030}{75,948} \times 100 = 31.6\%.$$

7. Half-Life
   Determine the intravascular survival or half-life by plotting either the cell-associated radioactivity (see calculation 6c) or the percent recovery (see calculation 6d) for the various blood samples collected on semilog graph paper.

   a. Plot the time of sample collection (hours) on the horizontal or linear (x) axis and the radioactivity or percent recovery on the vertical or logarithmic (y) axis.

   b. Draw a line of best fit through the points. The y-intercept is the recovery at zero time. The time interval between the recovery at zero time (eg, 32%) and half of the zero time recovery (eg, 16%) is the t½ or half-life. For example:

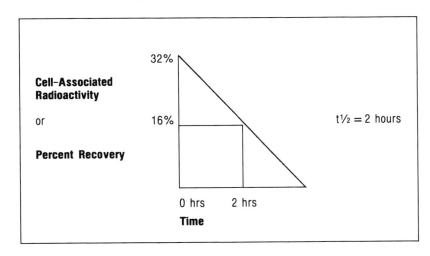

8. Specific activity
   The specific activity is the cpm/cell. This value is used in calculating the number of indium 111-labeled cells which have migrated into skin chambers (see section 6.2).

   a. Total cell-associated radioactivity injected: Multiply total radioactivity injected (see calculation 1) times the percent of all cell-associated radioactivity (see calculation 4).
      For example, if the total cpm injected is 500,000,000 and the percent of cell-associated radioactivity is 88.1%, then the total cell-associated cpm injected = 500,000,000 × 0.881 = 440,500,000.

b. Total number of cells injected: Multiply the granulocyte count, (eg 20,000/μL) times the total volume of the labeled cell suspension injected (eg, 5 mL or 5,000 μL).

Total cells injected = 20,000 × 5,000 = 100,000,000 or 1 × 10^8.

c. Specific activity =

$$\frac{\text{Total cell-assoc. cpm injected (see calculation 8a)}}{\text{Total cells injected (see calculation 8b)}}.$$

For example, if 1 × 10^8 cells were injected and the total cell-associated radioactivity was 440,500,000 then the specific activity =

$$\frac{440{,}500{,}000}{100{,}000{,}000} = 4.4 \text{ cpm/cell.}$$

References

Weiblen BJ, Forstrom L, McCullough J: Studies of the kinetics of indium 111-labeled granulocytes. *J Lab Clin Med* 94:246–255, 1979.

Thakur ML, Lavender JP, Arnot RN, et al: Indium 111-labeled autologous leukocytes in man. *J Nucl Med* 18:1014–1021, 1977.

Weiblen BJ, McCullough J, Forstrom LA, et al: Kinetics of indium 111-labeled granulocytes, in Thakur ML, Gottschalk A (eds): *Indium 111-labeled neutrophils, platelets, and lymphocytes*. New York, Trivirum Publishing Company, pp 23–32, 1980.

Thakur ML, Coleman RE, Welch MJ. Indium 111-labeled leukocytes for the localization of abscesses: Preparation, analysis, tissue distribution, and comparisons with gallium-67 citrate in dogs. *J Lab Clin Med* 89:217–221, 1977.

6.2 Skin Window Studies with Indium 111-Labeled Granulocytes

Materials

1. 10 mL evacuated serum tubes, sterile, silicon-coated
2. Tuberculin syringes
3. Centrifuge
4. Shaving cream
5. Safety razor
6. Betadine applicators
7. Alcohol swabs
8. Plastic custom-made blocks, sterile

a. Vacuum manifold block with three 8 mm bores

b. Chamber block

NOTE: If plexiglass plastic blocks are used, the poor thermal stability of that plastic requires that they be sterilized by gas autoclaving. Polycarbonate plastic blocks may be steam autoclaved.

9. Rubber serum stopper (plug O.D. 11 mm, sleeve O.D. 17 mm)

NOTE: Cut the top injection port sleeves off using a single-edge razor blade and the aluminum holding block made for this purpose.

10. Two velcro-elastic tourniquets

11. 250 W infrared lamp with porcelain receptacle with clamp for attaching unit to a ring stand or IV pole

12. Variable transformer suitable for 250 W service

13. Digital 9V electronic thermometer with remote sensing probe

14. Vacuum/pressure pump capable of sustaining continuous vacuum of 250 to 400 mm Hg suction pressure

15. Penlight flashlight

16. Forceps, sterile

17. Iris scissors, sterile

18. Surgical tape

a. 1 inch

b. 1/2 inch

19. Needles

a. 21 gauge

b. 27 gauge

20. 2 inch ace elastic wrap

21. Adaptic nonadherent dressing

22. 4 × 4 gauze, sterile

23. 12 × 75 mm borosilicate culture tubes

24. Automated cell counter or hemocytometer and microscope

25. Gamma counter

Reagent
1. 5% disodium edetate, (Na_2EDTA)

Method

Application of Chambers

1. Draw 30 mL blood from the donor and place in three 10 mL evacuated serum tubes. Cap the serum tubes and allow the blood to clot 45 to 60 minutes.

2. Centrifuge the tubes at 900 × g for 5 minutes. Pool serum (a minimum of 6 mL is required for the procedure). Centrifuge the serum a second time maintaining sterility.

3. Fill three 1 mL syringes with serum and refrigerate (4°C) with the remainder of serum.

4. Choose a fleshy site (away from the paths of long tendons) on the proximal volar forearm. If possible, avoid areas with visible surface veins.

5. Shave the arm of the donor if necessary.

6. Clean with betadine solution. Remove betadine with an alcohol swab.

Method for Skin Window Studies

7. Position the sterilized vacuum manifold block on the arm with two firmly applied elastic tourniquets, making certain the donor can bend the arm without difficulty and circulation is maintained (Figure 13–6).

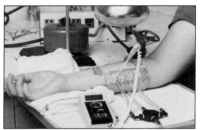

13–6 Apparatus positioned for blister formation: a) acrylic block with separate suction controls for each chamber attached to vacuum pump (not shown), b) thermometer with remote sensing probe, c) infrared lamp.

Notes _____

_____

_____

_____

_____

_____

_____

_____

8. Connect the infrared lamp into the variable transformer and position it about 10 inches over the vacuum block.

9. Place the thermometer probe into the hole in the block until it touches the donor's skin. Adjust the transformer until the skin temperature reaches about 32°C.

10. Begin suction at 250 mm Hg pressure by the gauge. The skin temperature should now be brought up to about 37°C by adjusting the transformer, and maintained at 37 ± 1°C until completion of the procedure. Avoid burning the skin by making certain the lamp is directly over the suction block and by placing gauze over any surrounding skin which is directly exposed to the light rays.

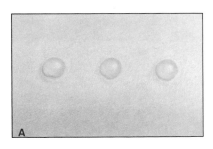

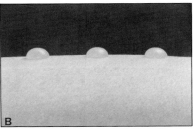

13-7 & 13-8 Appearance of well-formed blisters after removal of acrylic suction block [A) top view, B) side view].

11. Periodically monitor the formation of the blisters by placing a flashlight close to the top of the blister chamber and looking in the side. Typically, three clear, well-formed 8 mm diameter blisters will have formed in about 2 hours (Figures 13–7 and 13–8). Suction pressure may be varied to aid in blister formation. However, care must be taken not to increase it too rapidly or blisters may break.

Notes _____

_____

_____

_____

_____

_____

_____

_____

_____

_____

12. Turn off the pump. Remove all apparatus, being careful not to rupture blisters. Clean the surrounding area with alcohol swabs.

13. Using sterile forceps and iris scissors, gently cut the blisters at their perimeter and unroof the denuded dermis (Figures 13–9 and 13–10). Wipe off the excess fluid around the lesions with an alcohol swab taking care not to actually touch lesions.

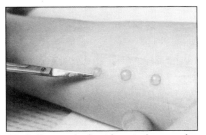

13-9 Removal of epidermis from each blister using iris scissors.

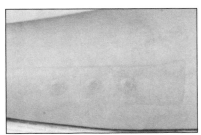

13-10 Denuded dermis at blister sites showing absence of bleeding.

Notes _____

_____

_____

_____

_____

_____

_____

_____

_____

_____

_____

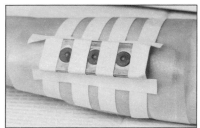

13-11 Placement of chamber block with rubber stoppers directly over lesions.

14. Align the sterile chamber block and three modified rubber stoppers with the visible indentations from the suction block on the donor's arm. Place the three modified rubber stoppers (injection ports) directly over the lesions (Figure 13–11).

Notes _____

_____

_____

_____

15. Put 1 inch tape across each end of the block and put several taut strips of 1/2 inch surgical tape over the top of the block in the spaces between chamber injection ports. Do not tape the entire circumference of the arm as this will cut off circulation. Run a 1/2 inch piece of tape down the length of the block on both sides to help prevent leakage.

16. Introduce an open 21 gauge needle as a vent into a chamber. Empty a serum-filled 1 mL tuberculin syringe into the chamber through a second needle. Remove venting needle. Fill all three chambers.

17. With the arm turned so the chamber is pointed to the side, carefully enter the septum of an injection port with needle pointed upward and withdraw 0.3 mL of air (Figure 13–12). This forms a vacuum in the chamber and helps to hold the block in position.

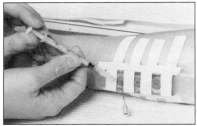

13-12 Technique for chamber injection or sampling using tuberculin syringe and second needle for venting.

Notes _____

_____

_____

_____

18. Check for leaks and make sure block feels securely attached to the arm. Wrap the site with the ace bandage (Figure 13–13).
   CAUTION: Do not wrap too tightly and instruct donor to loosen bandage if his/her hand begins to swell.

Notes _____

_____

_____

_____

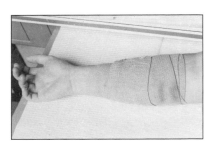

13-13 Securing chamber block to arm with elastic bandage for extended wear.

19. Inject the donor with indium 111-labeled granulocytes (see procedure 6.1).

■ Removal of Chambers

1. Remove the ace bandage. Instruct the donor to lay his arm on a table with the block accessible on the side of arm.

2. With an open 21 gauge needle pointed in an upward direction, carefully vent the first chamber.

3. With a tuberculin syringe and 27 gauge needle, carefully remove serum from the well by entering the chamber septum in a downward direction. Continue this procedure to empty the rest of the chambers, keeping fluids from each well separate. Place the fluid from each chamber in a 12 × 75 mm labeled tube containing 20 μL of 5% Na$_2$EDTA. Gently mix the tube.

4. Refill each chamber with 1 mL of fresh serum (see application procedure 16–18). Instruct the donor to gently shake his arm to facilitate rinsing.

5. Remove the serum as in the previous step and place in tubes labeled 1′, 2′, 3′ to denote rinse.

6. Cut the tape along the sides of the block and lift the block off gently (Figure 13–14).

Notes _____

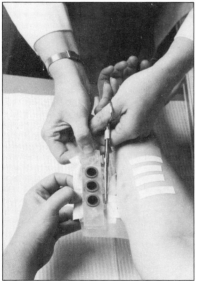

13–14 Removal of chamber block after final sampling is completed.

7. Place any extra fluid into the appropriate tube. The lesions should appear red but not bleeding. Remove the remaining tape.

8. Instruct the donor to gently wash lesions under running, lukewarm water. Cover the lesions with an adaptic nonadhering dressing, then with a 4 × 4 gauze sponge and secure the gauze with tape.

9. Remove the dressing after 24 hours. If the lesions look clean and reasonably dry after 24 hours, allow to crust over by being left open to the air.

■ **Sample Processing**

1. Perform a white blood cell count on the chamber fluid in duplicate (duplicates should be within 5% of each other). Record these counts in Column A of the data sheet (Figure 13–15) corresponding to the appropriate chamber.

Figure 13–15.

Data sheet for recording skin window sampling results.

INDIUM STUDIES DATA SHEET

Subject: _____

Skin Window Conditions: _____ 400 mm Hg pressure _____

White Cell Conditions: _____ 8 hour storage room temperature _____

Performance: _____ 3 good blisters (some leakage in #1 sample) _____

Ht: _____ in _____ cm   Blood Volume: _____ mL

Wt: _____ lbs _____ kg   WBC: _____ WBC/mm³

24-HOUR WBC COUNTS

Window #	A Raw Count $\times 10^3$/mm³	B Mean WBC $\times 10^6$/mL	C Volume mL	D Total WBC $\times 10^6$/tube	E Grand Total WBC $\times 10^6$/chamber
1	50.0 & 50.2	50.1	1.0	50.1	55.1
2	50.0 & 55.3	55.2	1.0	55.2	60.3
3	52.5 & 52.5	52.5	1.0	52.5	57.4
1'	5.0 & 5.0	5.0	1.0	5.0	
2'	5.1 & 5.1	5.1	1.0	5.1	
3'	4.9 & 4.9	4.9	1.0	4.9	

24-HOUR RADIOACTIVITY

Window #	F Count cpm/tube		G Mean cpm/tube	H Decay Corrected cpm/tube	I # Labeled WBC/tube	J # Labeled WBC/chamber
1	2,579	2,415	2,497	3,008	6,400	7,812
2	3,072	2,777	2,925	3,524	7,498	8,298
3	2,588	2,830	2,709	3,264	6,945	8,149
1'	559	543	551	664	1,412	
2'	315	308	312	376	800	
3'	494	445	470	566	1,204	

2. Calculate and record the mean value of the counts in Column B.

3. The total number of cells in each sample is derived as the product of the cell count (Column B) and the volume of chamber fluid (Column C). Record in Column D.

   For example: (See Row 1, Column D under heading "24-hour WBC counts") 50.1×10^6 WBC/mL $\times$ 1.0 mL = 50.1×10^6 WBC/tube.

4. Determine the total number of white blood cells per chamber for all samples (including rinses from a given chamber). This gives the total number of cells entering that chamber during the collection period. Record this value in Column E.

   For example: (See Row 1, Column E under heading "24-hour WBC counts") $50.1 + 5.0 \times 10^6 = 55.1 \times 10^6$.

5. Count the tubes twice with a gamma counter for 1.0 minute using the correct setting for indium 111. Count 1.0 mL of pre-study serum (or saline solution if serum is depleted) and set background to this number. Record the counts in Column F corresponding to the appropriate chamber.

6. Average the counts and record the mean value in Column G.

7. Correct for decay by calculating the difference in time between counting the samples for the kinetic study versus counting the skin chamber. Divide the mean cpm/tube (Column G) by the appropriate decay factor taken from Indium 111 Decay Factor Chart (Table 13–1), and record the value in Column H.

   For example: If the kinetic samples were counted at 12:30 a.m., June 12, and the skin chamber samples were counted at 6:30 p.m., June 12, the time elapsed would be 18 hours. See Table 13–1. Find 18 in the elapsed time column and note that the remaining activity is 0.83. Divide the mean cpm/tube by this decay correction to obtain the decay-corrected cpm/tube.

   (See Row 1, Column H under heading "24-hour radioactivity")

   $$\frac{2{,}497 \text{ cpm/tube}}{0.83} = 3{,}008 \text{ cpm/tube.}$$

8. Determine the specific activity (see procedure 6.1, calculation 8). Divide the decay-corrected radioactivity by the specific activity. Record value in Column I.

   For example: (See Row 1, Column I under heading "24-hour radioactivity")

   $$\frac{3{,}008 \text{ cpm/tube}}{0.47 \text{ cpm/WBC}} = 6{,}400 \text{ WBC/tube.}$$

9. Calculate the total labeled WBC/chamber for all samples (including rinses from a given chamber). This gives the total num-

Table 13-1.   INDIUM 111 DECAY FACTOR CHART

Elapsed Time (hr)	t½	Decay Factor (activity remaining)	Elapsed Time (hr)	t½	Decay Factor (activity remaining)
2	.030	.979	52	.776	.584
4	.060	.959	54	.806	.572
6	.090	.939	56	.836	.561
8	.119	.921	58	.866	.549
10	.149	.902	60	.896	.537
12	.179	.883	62	.925	.527
14	.209	.865	64	.955	.516
16	.239	.847	66	.985	.505
18	.269	.830	68	1.015	.495
20	.299	.813	70	1.045	.485
22	.328	.797	72	1.075	.475
24	.358	.780	74	1.104	.465
26	.388	.764	76	1.134	.455
28	.418	.749	78	1.164	.446
30	.448	.733	80	1.194	.437
32	.478	.718	82	1.224	.428
34	.507	.704	84	1.254	.420
36	.537	.687	86	1.284	.411
38	.567	.675	88	1.313	.403
40	.597	.661	90	1.343	.394
42	.627	.648	92	1.373	.386
44	.657	.634	94	1.403	.378
46	.687	.621	96	1.433	.370
48	.716	.605	98	1.463	.303
50	.746	.506	100	1.498	.355

NOTE: t½=67 hrs or 2.8 days

ber of labeled cells entering that chamber during the collection period. Record this value in Column J.

For example: (See Row 1, Column J under heading "24-hour radioactivity") 6,400 WBC/tube + 1,412 WBC/tube = 7,812 WBC/chamber.

References

Hellum KB, Solberg CO: Human leucocyte migration: Studies with an improved skin chamber technique. *Acta Path Microbiol Scand* 85:413–423, 1977.

McCullough J, Weiblen BJ, Fine D: Effects of storage of granulocytes on their fate in vivo. *Transfusion* 23:20–24, 1983.

Manufacturers' List

1. American Critical Care, McGraw Park, IL 60085
2. Amersham Corporation, 2636 S. Clearbrook Drive, Arlington Heights, IL 60005
3. Amicon, 24 Cherry Hill Drive, Danvers, MA 01923
4. Bio-Rad Laboratories, 2200 Wright Avenue, Richmond, CA 94804
5. Cel-Line Associates, P. O. Box 35, Newfield, NJ 08344
6. Cryoserve—Research Industries Corporation, Pharmaceutical Division, Salt Lake City, UT 84119
7. Cutter Biologicals, Berkeley, CA 94710
8. Difco Laboratories, P.O. 1058, Detroit, MI 48232
9. Fisher Scientific, 1600 W. Glenlake Avenue, P. O. Box 171, Itasca, IL 60143
10. Gibco, Grand Island Biological Company, 3175 Staley Road, Grand Island, NY 14072
11. Hamilton Company, Box 10030, Reno, NV 89510
12. Kallestad, 2000 National Bank Tower, Austin, TX 78701
13. Monoject, Division of Sherwood Medical, St. Louis, MO 63103
14. Pelfreez Biologicals, 9099 N. Deerbrook Trail, Brown Deer, WI 53209
15. Pharmacia Fine Chemicals, Piscataway, NJ 08854
16. Robbins Scientific Co., 1280 Space Park Way, Mountain View, CA 94043
17. Sigma Chemical Company, P. O. Box 14508, St. Louis, MO 63178
18. Winthrop Laboratories, 90 Park Avenue, New York, NY 10016
19. York Instruments, H.B. Manufacturing Company, 1035 Grayson Street, Berkeley, CA 94710

References

1. Doan CA: The recognition of a biologic differentiation in the white blood cells with a specific reference to blood transfusion. *JAMA* 86:1593–1597, 1926.

2. Dausset J, Nenna A: Presence d'une leuco-agglutinine dans le serum d'un cas d'agranulocytose chronique. *Compt Rend Soc Biol* 146:1539–1546, 1952.

3. Goudsmit R, van Loghem JJ: Studies on the occurrence of leukocyte-antibodies. *Vox Sang* 3:58–67, 1953.

4. Van Rood JJ, van Leeuwen A, Eernisse JG: Leukocyte antibodies in sera of pregnant women. *Vox Sang* 4:427–444, 1959.

5. Payne R, Rolfs MR: Fetomaternal leukocyte incompatibility. *J Clin Invest* 37:1756–1763, 1958.

6. Moeschlin S, Wagner K: Agranulocytosis due to the occurrence of leukocyte-agglutinins (pyramidon and cold agglutinins). *Acta Hematol* 8:29–41, 1952.

7. Payne R, Rolfs MR: Further observation on leukoagglutinin transfusion reactions, with special reference to leukoagglutinin transfusion reactions in women. *Am J Med* 29:449–458, 1960.

8. Terasaki PI, Bernoco D, Park MS, et al: Microdroplet testing for HLA-A, -B, -C, and -D antigens. Am J Clin Pathol 69:103–120, 1978.

9. Lalezari P, Radel E: Neutrophil-specific antigens: Immunology and clinical significance. *Semin Hematol* 11:281–290, 1974.

10. Lalezari P, Nussbaum M, Gelman S, et al: Neonatal neutropenia due to maternal isoimmunization. *Blood* 15:236–243, 1960.

11. Lalezari P, Bernard JE: An isologous antigen-antibody reaction with human neutrophils related to neonatal neutropenia. *J Clin Invest* 45:1741–1750, 1966.

12. Lalezari P, Murphy GB, Allen FH: NB1, a new neutrophil antigen involved in the pathogenesis of neonatal neutropenia. *J Clin Invest* 50:1108–1115, 1971.

13. Lalezari P, Thalenfeld B, Weinstein WJ: The third neutrophil antigen, in Terasaki PI (ed): *Histocompatibility Testing, 1970.* Baltimore: Williams and Wilkins Co., 1970, pp 319–322.

14. Lalezari P: Alloimmune neonatal neutropenia and neutrophil-specific antigens. *Vox Sang* 46:415–417, 1984.

15. Boxer LA, Yokoyama M, Lalezari P: Isoimmune neonatal neutropenia. *J Pediatr* 80:783–787, 1972.

16. Chusid MJ, Pisciotta AV, Duquesnoy RJ, et al: Congenital neutropenia: Studies of pathogenesis. *Am J Hematol* 8:315–324, 1980.

17. Lalezari P: Neutrophil specific antigens: Their relationship to neonatal and acquired neutropenias with comments on the possible role of organ specific alloantigens in organ transplantation. *Transplant Proc* 9:1881–1886, 1977.

18. Minchinton RM, Waters AH: The occurrence and significance of neutrophil antibodies. *Br J Haematol* 56:521–528, 1984.

19. Boxer LA, Greenberg S, Boxer GJ, et al: Autoimmune neutropenia. *N Engl J Med* 293:748–753, 1975.

20. Von dem Borne AEGKr, van der Plas-van Dalen C, Engelfriet CP: Immunofluorescence antiglobulin test, in McMillan R (ed): *Immune Cytopenias.* New York: Churchill Livingstone, 1983, pp 106–127.

21. Madyastha PR, Fudenberg HH, Glassman AB, et al: Autoimmune neutropenia in early infancy: A review. *Ann Clin Lab Sci* 12:356–367, 1982.

22. Priest JR, Ramsay NKC, Clay ME, et al: Transient autoimmune neutropenia due to anti-NA1 antibody. *Am J Pediatr Hematol Oncol* 2:195–199, 1980.

23. Yomtovian R, Kline W, Press C, et al: Severe pulmonary hypersensitivity associated with passive transfusion of a neutrophil specific antibody. *Lancet* 1:244–246, 1984.

24. McCullough J, Weiblen BJ, Clay ME, et al: Effect of leukocyte antibodies on the fate in vivo of indium-111–labeled granulocytes. *Blood* 58:164–170, 1981.

25. McCullough JJ, Clay ME, Richards K, et al: Leukocyte antibodies: Their effect on the fate in vivo of indium-111 labeled granulocytes, Abstracted. *Blood* 60:80a, 1982.

26. Boxer LA, Stossel TP: Effects of anti-human neutrophil antibodies in vitro: Quantitative studies. *J Clin Invest* 53:1534–1545, 1974.

27. Cotter TG, Spears P, Henson PM: A monoclonal antibody inhibiting human neutrophil chemotaxis and degranulation. *J Immunol* 127:1355–1360, 1981.

28. Cotter TG, Keeling PJ, Henson PM: A monoclonal antibody inhibiting fMLP-induced chemotaxis of human neutrophils. *J Immunol* 127:2241–2245, 1981.

29. McCullough J, Clay ME, Priest JR, et al: A comparison of methods for detecting leukocyte antibodies in autoimmune neutropenia. *Transfusion* 21:483–492, 1981.

30. Dausset J, Nenna A, Brecy H: Leukoagglutinin. V. Leukoagglutinins in chronic idiopathic or symptomatic pancytopenia and in paroxysmal nocturnal hemoglobinuria. *Blood* 9:696–720, 1954.

31. Lalezari P: A new technic for the separation of human leukocytes. *Blood* 19:109–114, 1962.

32. Greenwalt TJ, Polka R: Gum acacia for preparing suspensions on leukocytes. *Am J Clin Pathol* 33:358–361, 1960.

33. Engelfriet CP, von Loghem JJ: Studies on leucocyte iso- and auto-antibodies. *Br J Haematol* 7:223–238, 1961.

34. Lalezari P, Weinstein WJ, Thalenfeld B: A rapid method for preparation of human leukocytes, in Terasaki PI (ed): *Histocompatibility Testing 1970*. Copenhagen: Munksgaard, 1970, pp 631–632.

35. Boyum A: Isolation of mononuclear cells and granulocytes from blood. Isolation of mononuclear cells by one centrifugation and of granulocytes by combining centrifugation and sedimentation at 1 g. *Scand J Clin Lab Invest* 21(suppl 97):77–89, 1968.

36. English D, Anderson BR: Single-step separation of red blood cells, granulocytes, and mononuclear leukocytes on discontinuous density gradients of Ficoll-Hypaque. *J Immunol Methods* 5:249–252, 1974.

37. Ferrante A, Thong YH: A rapid one-step procedure for purification of mononuclear and polymorphonuclear leukocytes from human blood using a modification of the Hypaque-Ficoll technique. *J Immunol Methods* 24:389–393, 1978.

38. Ferrante A, Thong YH: Optimal conditions for simultaneous purification of mononuclear and polymorphonuclear leukocytes from human blood by the Hypaque-Ficoll method. *J Immunol Methods* 36:109–117, 1980.

39. Madyastha P, Madyastha KR, Wade T, et al: An improved method for rapid layering of Ficoll-Hypaque double density gradients suitable for granulocyte separation. *J Immunol Methods* 48:281–286, 1982.

40. Yust I, Smith RW, Wunderlich JR, et al: Temporary inhibition of antibody-dependent, cell-mediated cytotoxicity by pretreatment of human attacking cells with ammonium chloride. *J Immunol* 4:1170–1172, 1976.

41. Dooley DC, Takahashi T: The effect of osmotic stress on the function of the human granulocyte. *Exp Hematol* 9:731–741, 1981.

42. Segal AW, Fortunato A, Herd T: A rapid single centrifugation step method for the separation of erythrocytes, granulocytes and mononuclear cells on continuous density gradients of Percoll. *J Immunol Methods* 32:209–214, 1980.

43. Berger CL, Edelson RL: Comparison of lymphocyte function after isolation by Ficoll-Hypaque flotation or elutriation. *J Invest Dermatol* 73:231–235, 1979.

44. Kurnick JT, Ostberg L, Stegagno M, et al: A rapid method for the separation of functional lymphoid cell populations of human or animal origin on PVP-silica (Percoll) density gradients. *Scand J Immunol* 10:563–573, 1979.

45. Roth JA, Kaeberle ML: Isolation of neutrophils and eosinophils from the peripheral blood of cattle and comparison of the functional activities. *J Immunol Methods* 45:153–164, 1981.

46. Bruch C, Kovecs P, Ruber E, et al: Studies on the inhibitory effect of granulocytes on human granulopoiesis in agar cultures. *Exp Hematol* 6:337–345, 1978.

47. Pertoft H, Rubin K, Kjellen L, et al: The viability of cells grown or centrifuged in a new density gradient medium, Percoll. *Exp Cell Res* 110:449–457, 1977.

48. Hjorth R, Jonasson AK, Vretblad P: A rapid method for purification of human granulocytes using Percoll. A comparison with dextran sedimentation. *J Immunol Methods* 43:95–101, 1981.

49. Dooley DC, Simpson JS, Meryman HT: Isolation of large numbers of fully viable human neutrophils: A preparative technique using Percoll density gradient centrifugation. *Exp Hematol* 10:591–599, 1982.

50. Redl H, Hammerschmidt DE, Schlag G. Augmentation by platelets of granulocyte aggregation in response to chemotaxins: Studies utilizing an improved cell preparation technique. *Blood* 61:125–131, 1983.

51. Dausset J: Iso-leuco-anticorps. *Acta Haematol* (Basel) 20:156–166, 1958.

52. Terasaki PI, McClelland JB: Microdroplet assay of human serum cytotoxins. *Nature* (London) 204:998–1000, 1964.

53. Waalford RL, Gallagher R, Sjaarda JR: Serological typing of human lymphocytes with immune serum obtained after homografting. *Science* 144:868–870, 1964.

54. Lalezari P, Bernard GE: Improved leukocyte antibody detection with prolonged incubation. *Vox Sang* 9:664–672, 1964.

55. Lalezari P, Jiang A, Lee S: A microagglutination technique for detection of leukocyte agglutinins, in Ray JG, Hare DB, Pederson PD, et al (eds): *NIAID Manual: A Tissue Typing Technique.* US Dept of Health, Education, and Welfare publication No. (NIH) 77–545, pp 4–6, 1976.

56. Lalezari P, Pryce SC: Detection of neutrophil and platelet antibodies in immunologically induced neutropenia and thrombocytopenia, in Rose NR, Friedmann H (eds): *Manual of Clinical Immunology.* Washington, DC: Am Soc Microbiol, 1980, pp 744–749.

57. Lalezari P: Neutrophil antigens: Immunology and clinical implications, in Greenwalt TJ, Jamieson GA (eds): *The Granulocyte: Function and Clinical Utilization.* Progress in Clinical and Biological Research, New York: Alan R. Liss, 1977, pp 209–225.

58. Lalezari P: Alloantigens specific to blood polymorphonuclear neutrophils, in Cohen E, Singal D (eds): *Non-HLA Antigens in Health, Aging, and Malignancy.* Progress in Clinical and Biological Research, New York: Alan R. Liss, 1983, pp 23–30.

59. Verheugt FWA, von dem Borne AEGKr, van Noord-Bokhorst JC, et al: Serological, immunochemical and immunocytological properties of antibodies. *Vox Sang* 35:294–303, 1978.

60. Engelfriet CP, Tetteroo PAT, van der Veen JPW, et al: Granulocyte-specific antigens and methods for their detection, in McCullough J, Sandler SG (eds): *Advances in Immunobiology: Blood Cell Antigens and Bone Marrow Transplantation.* Progress in Clinical and Biological Research, New York: Alan R. Liss, 1984, pp 121–154.

61. Lalezari P, Petrosova M, Jiang AF: NB2, an allele of NB1 neutrophil specific antigen: Relationship to 9a, abstracted. *Transfusion* 22:433, 1982.

62. Severson CD, Greazel NA, Thompson JS: Micro-capillary agglutination. *J Immunol Methods* 4:369–380, 1974.

63. Thompson JS, Severson CD: Granulocyte antigens, in Bell CA (ed): *A Seminar on Antigens on Blood Cells and Body Fluid.* Washington, DC: American Association of Blood Banks, 1980, pp 151–187.

64. Thompson JS: Antileukocyte capillary agglutinating antibody in pre- and post-transplantation sera, in Rose NR, Friedman H (eds): *Manual of Clinical Immunology.* Washington DC: Am Soc Microbiol, 1976, pp 868–873.

65. Smith WK, Mold JW, Tseng SL, et al: Microcapillary agglutination assay for detection of specific antileukocyte reactivity in neutropenic patients. *Am J Hematol* 7:329–340, 1979.

66. Thompson JS, Jackson D, Greazel NA, et al: Antileukocyte antibodies in postpartum and renal transplant subjects. *Transplantation* 21:85–93, 1976.

67. Thompson JS, Severson CD, Parmely MJ, et al: "Pulmonary hypersensitivy" reactions induced by transfusion of non-HL-A leukoagglutinins. *N Engl J Med* 284:1120–1125, 1971.

68. Hasegawa T, Graw RG, Terasaki PI: A microgranulocyte cytotoxicity test. *Transplantation* 15:492–498, 1973.

69. Engelfriet CP: Cytotoxic antibodies against leukocytes, in Amos DB, van Rood JJ (eds): *Histocompatibility Testing* 1970. Copenhagen: Munksgaard, 1965, pp 245–250.

70. Caplan SN, Berkman EM, Babior BM: Cytotoxins against a granulocyte antigen system: Detection by a new method employing cytochalasin-B-treated cells. *Vox Sang* 33:206–211, 1977.

71. Drew SI, Bergh O, McClelland J, et al: Antigenic specificities detected on papainized human granulocytes by microgranulocytotoxicity. *Transplant Proc* 9:639–645, 1977.

72. Hasegawa T, Bergh OJ, Mickey MR, et al: Preliminary human granulocyte specificities. *Transplant Proc* 7(suppl 1):75–80, 1975.

73. Korinkova P, Vorlicek J, Majsky A: A study of granulocyte cytotoxins and detection of granulocyte allospecific antigens. *Transfusion* 22:379–383, 1982.

74. Takasugi M: Improved fluorochromatic cytotoxic test. *Transplantation* 12:148–151, 1971.

75. Lizak GE, Grumet FC: A new micromethod for the in vitro detection of antiplatelet antibodies: C-FDA thrombocytotoxicity. *Hum Immunol* 1:87–96, 1980.

76. Thompson JS, Overlin VL, Herbick JM, et al: New granulocyte antigens demonstrated by microgranulocytotoxicity assay. *J Clin Invest* 65:1431–1439, 1980.

77. Blaschke J, Goeken NE, Thompson JS, et al: Acquired agranulocytosis with granulocyte specific cytotoxic autoantibody. *Am J Med* 66:862–866, 1979.

78. Drew SI, Carter BM, Guidera D, et al: Further aspects of microgranulocytotoxicity. *Transfusion* 19:434–443, 1979.

79. Drew SI, Terasaki PI: Autoimmune cytotoxic granulocyte antibodies in normal persons and various diseases. *Blood* 52:941–952, 1978.

80. Calabresi P, Edwards EA, Schilling RF: Fluorescent antiglobulin studies in leukopenic and related disorders. *J Clin Invest* 38:2091–2100, 1959.

81. Verheugt FWA, von dem Borne AEGKr, Decary S, et al: The detection of granulocyte alloantibodies with an indirect immunofluorescence test. *Br J Haematol* 36:533–544, 1977.

82. Verheugt FWA, von dem Borne AEGKr, van Noord-Bokhorst JC, et al: Autoimmune granulocytopenia: The detection of granulocyte autoantibodies with the immunofluorescence test. *Br J Haematol* 39:339–350, 1978.

83. Zaroulis CG, Jaramillo S: A microimmunofluorescent assay to detect human granulocyte antigens and antibodies. *Am J Hematol* 10:65–73, 1981.

84. Press C, Kline WE, Clay ME, et al: A microtiter modification of granulocyte immunofluorescence. *Vox Sang* 49:110–113, 1985.

85. Boxer GJ, Boxer MA, Boxer LA: The identification of antiplatelet and antineutrophil antibodies by ^{125}I-staphylococcal protein A, in McMillan R (ed): *Immune Cytopenias*. New York: Churchill Livingstone, 1983, pp 87–105.

86. Sjoquist J, Meloun B, Hjelm H: Protein A isolated from *Staphylococcus aureus* after digestion with lyfostaphin. *Eur J Biochem* 29:572–578, 1972.

87. McCallister JA, Boxer LA, Baehner RL: The use and limitation of labeled staphylococcal protein A for study of antineutrophil antibodies. *Blood* 54:1330–1337, 1979.

88. Gooding JW: Use of staphylococcal protein A as an immunological reagent. *J Immunol Methods* 20:241–253, 1978.

89. Stossel TP: Immune-mediated neutrophil destruction, in Bell CA (ed): *A Seminar on Immune-mediated Cell Destruction*. Washington, DC: American Association of Blood Banks, 1981, pp 199–208.

90. Harmon DC, Weitzman SA, Stossel TP: A staphylococcal slide test for detection of antineutrophil antibodies. *Blood* 56:64–69, 1980.

91. Harmon DC, Weitzman SA, Stossel TP: A slide test for detecting neutrophil associated complement component. *Transfusion* 23:131–134, 1983.

92. Lazar GS, Gaidulis L, Henke M, et al: A sensitive screening method of detecting anti-granulocyte antibodies employing radiolabeled staphylococcal protein A. *J Immunol Methods* 68:1–9, 1984.

93. Parmley RT, Crist WM, Regal AH, et al: Congenital dysgranulopoietic neutropenia: Clinical, serologic, ultrastructural and in vitro proliferative characteristics. *Blood* 56:465–475, 1980.

94. Blumfelder T, Logue G: Human IgG antigranulocyte antibodies: Comparison of detection by quantitative antiglobulin and by binding of ^{125}I-staph protein A. *Am J Hematol* 11:77–84, 1981.

95. Hsu SM, Raine L: Protein A, avidin and biotin in immunohistochemistry. *J Histochem Cytochem* 29:1349–1353, 1981.

96. Guesdon J, Ternynck T, Avrameaus S: The use of avidin-biotin interaction in immunoenzymatic techniques. *J Histochem Cytochem* 27:1131–1138, 1979.

97. Bayer E, Skutelsky E, Wilchek M: The avidin-biotin complex in affinity cytochemistry. *Methods Enzymol* 62:308–315, 1979.

98. Hsu SM, Raine L: Versatility of biotin-labeled lectins and avidin-biotin-peroxidase complex for localization of carbohydrate in tissue sections. *J Histochem Cytochem* 30:157–161, 1982.

99. Biotin-Avidin Immunoassays. *Immu-News: Cooper Biomedical Technical Newsletter on Immunology and Research and Products.* Marketing Department, Scientific Division, Cooper Biomedical, Malvern, PA, 1983, 2:3–4.

100. Henke M, Yonemoto LM, Lazar GS, et al: Visual detection of granulocyte surface antigens using the avidin-biotin complex. *J Histochem Cytochem* 32:712–716, 1984.

101. Engvall E, Perlmann P: Enzyme-linked immunosorbent assay (ELISA). Quantitative assay of immunoglobulin G. *Immunochem* 8:871–874, 1971.

102. Alosi RM, Dowd JC: An ELISA method for detecting unexpected antibodies. *Am J Med Tech* 47:913–918, 1981.

103. Gudino M, Miller WV: Application of the enzyme-linked immunospecific assay (ELISA) for the detection of platelet antibodies. *Blood* 57:32–37, 1981.

104. Tamerius JD, Curd JG, Tani P, et al: An enzyme-linked immunosorbent assay for platelet compatibility testing. *Blood* 62:744–749, 1983.

105. Schiffer CA, Young V: Detection of platelet antibodies using a microenzyme-linked immunosorbent assay (ELISA). *Blood* 61:311–317, 1983.

106. Mannoni P, Janowska-Wiezzorek A, Turner AR, et al: Monoclonal antibodies against human granulocytes and myeloid differentiation antigens. *Hum Immunol* 5:309–323, 1982.

107. Rustagi PK, Currie MS, Logue GL: Complement-activating antineutrophil antibody in systemic lupus erythematosus. *Am J Med* 78:971–977, 1985.

108. Cines DB, Pessaro F, Guerry D, et al: Granulocyte-associated IgG in neutropenic disorders. *Blood* 59:124–132, 1982.

109. Logue GL, Kurlander R, Pepe P, et al: Antibody-dependent lymphocyte-mediated granulocyte cytotoxicity in man. *Blood* 51:97–108, 1978.

110. Bom-van Noorloos AA, Pegels HG, van Oers RHJ, et al: Proliferation of T cells with killer-cell activity in two patients with neutropenia and recurrent infections. *N Engl J Med* 302:933–937, 1980.

111. Horwitz DA, Bakke AC: An Fc receptor-bearing third population of human mononuclear cells with cytotoxic and regulatory function. *Immunol Today* 5:148–153, 1984.

112. Roitt IM: *Essential Immunology.* 5th ed. St Louis: Mosby, 1984, p 369.

113. Fuson EW, Hubbard RA, Sugantharaj DG, et al: Antibody-dependent cell-mediated cytotoxicity: Effectors, signals and mechanisms. *Surv Immunol Res* 2:327–340, 1983.

114. Logue GL, Huang AT, Shimm DS: Failure of splenectomy in Felty's syndrome: The role of antibodies supporting granulocyte lysis by lymphocytes. *N Engl J Med* 304:580–583, 1981.

115. Richards K, Sadrzadeh SMH, Clay M, et al: Antibody-dependent lymphocyte-mediated granulocytotoxicity (ADLG) for the detection of granulocyte antibodies. *J Immunol Methods* 63:93–102, 1983.

116. Von dem Borne AEGKr, Verheugt FWA, Oosterhof E, et al: A simple immunofluorescence test for the detection of platelet antibodies. *Br J Haematol* 39:195–207, 1978.

117. Cline MJ, Opelz G, Saxon A, et al: Autoimmune panleukopenia. *N Engl J. Med* 295:1489–1493, 1976.

118. Nusbacher J, MacPhearson JL, Gore I, et al: Inhibition of granulocyte erythrophagocytosis by HLA antisera. *Blood* 53:350–357, 1979.

119. Miller ME, Boxer LA, Kawaoka EJ, et al: Cell elastimetry in the detection of antineutrophil antibodies. *Blood* 57:22–24, 1981.

120. Cline MJ, Golde WH: Immune suppression of hematopoiesis. *Am J Med* 64:301–310, 1978.

121. Starkebaum G, Arend WP: Neutrophil-binding immunoglobulin G in systemic lupus erythematosus. *J Clin Invest* 64:902–912, 1979.

122. Starkebaum G, Singer JW, Arend WP: Humoral and cellular immune mechanisms of neutropenia in patients with Felty's syndrome. *Clin Exp Immunol* 39:307–314, 1980.

123. Weitzman SA, Desmond MC, Stossel TP: Antigenic modulation and turnover in human polymorphonuclear leukocytes. *J Clin Invest* 64:321–325, 1979.

124. Logue GL: Immune neutropenia, in McCullough J, Sandler SG (eds): *Advances in Immunobiology: Blood Cell Antigens and Bone Marrow Transplantation.* Progress in Clinical and Biological Research, New York: Alan R. Liss, 1984, pp 155–165.

125. Minchinton RM, Waters AH, Malpas JS, et al: Platelet- and granulocyte-specific antibodies after allogeneic and autologous bone marrow grafts. *Vox Sang* 46:125–135, 1984.

126. Richman CM: Prolonged preservation of human granulocytes. *Transfusion* 23:508–511, 1983.

127. Van Oss CJ: Cryopreservation of phagocytes. *J Reticuloendothel Soc* 24:33–40, 1978.

128. Meryman HT, Howard J: Cryopreservation of granulocytes, in Greenwalt TJ, Jamieson GA (eds): *The Granulocyte: Function and Clinical Utilization.* Progress in Clinical and Biological Research, New York: Alan R. Liss, 1977, pp 193–201.

129. Boonlayangoor P, Telischi M, Boonlayangoor S, et al: Cryopreservation of human granulocytes: Study of granulocyte function and ultrastructure. *Blood* 56:237–245, 1980.

130. Valeri CR: The current state of platelet and granulocyte cryopreservation. *CRC Crit Rev Clin Lab Sci* 14(1):21–74, 1981.

131. Roos D, Voetman AA, Meerhof LJ. Functional activity of enucleated human polymorphonuclear leukocytes. *J Cell Biol* 97:368–377, 1983.

132. Voetman AA, Bot AAM, Roos D: Cryopreservation of enucleated human neutrophils (PMN cytoplasts). *Blood* 63:234–237, 1984.

133. Van der Veen JPW, Miedema F, Goldschmeding R, et al: Neutropenia in chronic Tγ lymphocytosis: Exploration of the possible causes, in van der Veen JPW (ed): *Immunological Aspects of Chronic Neutropenia,* thesis. Amsterdam, 1985, pp 85–109.

134. Helmerhorst FM, van Oss CJ, Bruynes ECE, et al: Elution of granulocyte and platelet antibodies. *Vox Sang* 43:196–204, 1982.

135. Edwards JM, Moulds JJ, Judd WJ: Chloroquine dissociation of antigen-antibody complexes. *Transfusion* 22:59–61, 1982.

136. Blumberg N, Masel D, Mayer T, et al: Removal of HLA-A,B antigens from platelets. *Blood* 63:448–450, 1984.

137. Nordhagen R, Flaathen ST: Chloroquine removal of HLA antigens from platelets for the platelet immunofluorescence test. *Vox Sang* 48:156–159, 1985.

138. Minchinton RM, Waters AH: Chloroquine stripping of HLA antigens from neutrophils without removal of neutrophil-specific antigens. *Br J Haematol* 57:703–706, 1984.

139. Young GAR, Vincent PC: Drug-induced agranulocytosis. *Clin Hematol* 9:483–504, 1980.

140. Weitzman SA, Stossel TP: Drug-induced immunological neutropenia. *Lancet* 1:1068–1072, 1978.

141. Thompson JS, Herbick JM, Klassen LW, et al: Studies on levamisole-induced agranulocytosis. *Blood* 56:388–396, 1980.

142. Moeschlin S: Immunological granulocytopenia and agranulocytosis. *Le Sang* 26:32–51, 1955.

143. Eisner EV, Carry RM, MacKinney AA: Quinidine-induced agranulocytosis. *JAMA* 238:884–886, 1977.

144. Bilezkian SB, Laleli Y, Tsang M, et al: Immunological reactions involving leukocytes. III. Agranulocytosis induced by antithyroid drugs. *Johns Hopkins Med J* 138:124–129, 1976.

145. Lawson AA, McArdele T, Ghosh S: Cephradine-associated immune neutropenia. *N Engl J Med* 312:651, 1985.

146. Rouveix B, Lassoude K, Vittecoq D, et al: Neutropenia due to B lactamine antibodies. *Br J Med* 287:1832–1834, 1983.

147. Boxer LA: Immune neutropenias: Clinical and biological implications. *Am J Pediatr Hematol Oncol* 3:89–96, 1981.

148. Van Beek RJJ, Bieger R, den Ottolander GJ: Reversible severe anaemia and granulocytopenia caused by procainamide. *Scand J Haematol* 21:150–152, 1978.

149. Drew SI, Carter BM, Nathanson TS, et al: Levamisole-associated neutropenia and autoimmune granulocytotoxins. *Ann Rheum Dis* 39:59–63, 1980.

150. Pisciotta AV, Cronkite C: Aprindine-induced agranulocytosis: Evidence for immunologic mechanism. *Arch Intern Med* 143:241–243, 1983.

151. Berkman EM, Orlan JB, Wolfsdorf J: An anti-neutrophil antibody associated with a propylthiouracil-induced lupus-like syndrome. *Transfusion* 23:135–138, 1983.

152. Van Leeuwen EF, Engelfriet CP, von dem Borne AEGKr: Studies on quinine- and quinidine-dependent antibodies against platelets and their reaction with platelets in the Bernard Soulier syndrome. *Br J Haematol* 51:551–560, 1982.

153. Yomtovian R, Kline W, Press C, et al: Evidence for granulocyte antibody activity in two cases of procainamide-associated neutropenia, abstracted. *Blood* 64(suppl 1):92a, 1984.

154. Lalezari P, Murphy GB: Cold reacting leukocyte agglutinins and their significance, in Curtoni ES, Mattinuz PL, Tosi RM (eds):

Histocompatibility Testing, 1967. Baltimore: Williams and Wilkins Co., 1967, pp 421–427.

155. Markenson AL, Lalezari P, Markenson JA, et al: *Proc 18th Congr Am Soc Hematol,* Dallas, 1975, p 194.

156. Lalezari P, Bernard G: Studies on human leukocyte antigens. *Proc 9th Congr Eur Soc Haematol,* Lisbon. New York: S Karger, 1963, pp 1084–1087.

157. Lalezari P: Biological roles of tissue-specific and systemic alloantigens, in McCullough J, Sandler SG (eds): *Advances in Immunobiology: Blood Cell Antigens and Bone Marrow Transplantation.* Progress in Clinical and Biological Research, New York: Alan R. Liss, 1984, pp 55–75.

158. Dunstan RA, Simpson MB, Knowles RW, et al: Absence of ABH antigens on human neutrophils, abstracted. *Blood* 64:84a, 1984.

159. Dunstan RA, Simpson MB: Status of major red blood group antigens on human neutrophils, monocytes and lymphocytes, abstracted. *Blood* 64:84a, 1984.

160. Gaidulis L, Branch DR, Lazar GS, et al: Failure to detect the red cell antigens A, B, D, U, Ge, Jk3 and Yt^a on granulocytes by direct measurement using I–125 staphylococcal protein or avidin-biotin-complex assay, abstracted. *Blood* 64:85a, 1984.

161. Kelton JG, Bebenek G. Granulocytes do not have surface ABO antigens. *Transfusion* 25:567–569, 1985.

162. Cook KM: Distribution of HL-A antigens on blood cells. *Tissue Antigens* 4:202–209, 1974.

163. Thorsby E: HL-A antigens on human granulocytes studied with cytotoxic iso-antisera obtained by skin grafting. *Scand J Haematol* 6:119–127, 1969.

164. Clay M, Kline W, McCullough J: The frequency of granulocyte-specific antibodies in post partum serum and a family study of the 6B antigen. *Transfusion* 24:252–255, 1984.

165. Starkebaum G, Arend WP, Nardella FA, et al: Characterization of immune complexes and immunoglobulin G antibodies reactive with neutrophils in the sera of patients with Felty's syndrome. *J Lab Clin Med* 96:238–251, 1980.

166. Caligaris-Cappio F, Camussi G, Gavisto F: Idiopathic neutropenia with normal cellular bone marrow: An immune-complex disease. *Br J Haematol* 43:595–605, 1979.

167. Caligaris-Cappio F, Camussi G, Novarino A, et al. Immune-complexes (IC) in idiopathic neutropenia. *Scand J Haematol* 27:311–322, 1981.

168. Rustagi PK, Currie MS, Logue GL: Activation of human complement by immunoglobulin G antigranulocyte antibody. *J Clin Invest* 70:1137–1147, 1982.

169. Fudenberg HH, Rosenfield RE, Wasserman LR: Unusual specificity of auto-antibody in auto-immune hemolytic disease. *Mt Sinai J Med* 25:324–328, 1958.

170. Issitt PD, Zellner DC, Rolih SD, et al: Autoantibodies mimicking alloantibodies. *Transfusion* 17:531–538, 1977.

171. Clay ME, Kline WE: Neutrophil antibodies: Detection and clinical application. *Am J Med Tech* 477:805–811, 1981.

172. Lalezari P: Autoimmune neutropenia. *Vox Sang* 46:418–420, 1984.

173. Lalezari P, Jiang AF, Yegen L, et al: Chronic autoimmune neutropenia due to anti-NA2 antibody. *N Engl J Med* 293:744–747, 1975.

174. Huang ST, Lin J, McGowan EI, et al: NB2, a new allele of NB1 antigen involved in febrile transfusion reaction, abstracted. *Transfusion* 22:426, 1982.

175. Verheugt FWA: *Neutrophil antigens and antibodies*, thesis. Amsterdam, 1977.

176. Schacter B, Preis P, Kadushin JM, et al: Family studies of neutrophil alloantigens in bone marrow transplantation. *Tissue Antigens* 16:267–273, 1980.

177. Schacter B, Kadushin J, Hsieh K: Neutrophil antigens: Population and family studies in Caucasians and blacks. *Hum Immunol* 1:280, 1980.

178. Kline WE, Press C, Uhlich A, et al: The relationship between neutrophil specific antigens NA2 and NC1, abstracted. *Transfusion* 24:322, 1984.

179. Verheugt FWA, von dem Borne AEGKr, van Noord-Bokhorst JC, et al: ND1, a new neutrophil granulocyte antigen. *Vox Sang* 35:13–17, 1978.

180. Claas FHJ, Langerak J, Sabbe LJM, et al: NE1, a new neutrophil specific antigen. *Tissue Antigens* 13:129–134, 1979.

181. Helmerhorst FM, Claas FHJ, van Dalen C, et al: Neutrophil specific antigen NE1 is not the antithetical allele of ND1. *Tissue Antigens* 18:139–140, 1981.

182. Van Rood JJ, van Leeuwen A, Schippers AMJ: Leukocyte groups, the normal lymphocyte transfer test and homograft sensitivity, in Amos DB, van Rood JJ (eds): *Histocompatibility Testing*. Copenhagen: Munksgaard, 1965, pp 37–50.

183. Mahmoud AF, Kellermeyer RW, Warren KS: Monospecific antigranulocyte sera against human neutrophils, eosinophils, basophils and myeloblasts. *Lancet* 2:1163–1166, 1974.

184. Thompson JS, Overlin V, Severson CD, et al: Demonstration of granulocyte, monocyte and endothelial cell antigens by double fluorochromatic microcytotoxicity testing. *Transplant Proc* 12(suppl 1):26–31, 1980.

185. Berroche L, Maupin B, Hervier P: Mise en évidence des antigenes A et B dans les leucocytes humains par des épreuves d'absorption et d'elution. *Vox Sang* 5:82–83, 1955.

186. Renton PH, Hancock JA: Uptake of A and B antigens by transfused group O erythrocytes. *Vox Sang* 7:33–38, 1962.

187. Lewis JH, Draude J, Kuhns WJ: Coating of "O" platelets with A and B blood group substances. *Vox Sang* 5:434–441, 1960.

188. McCullough J, Clay M, Hurd D, et al: Studies of the in vivo significance of blood group ABH antigens on granulocytes, abstracted. *Blood* 66:90a, 1985.

189. Karhi KK, Andersson LC, Vuopio P, et al: Expression of blood group A antigens in human bone marrow. *Blood* 57:147–151, 1981.

190. Dausset J: Leuco-agglutinins. IV. Leuco-agglutinins and blood transfusion. *Vox Sang* 4:190–198, 1954.

191. Metzgar RS, Zmijewski CM, Siegler HF: A comparison of the leukocyte agglutination and mixed agglutination techniques to detect human tissue antigens. *Transplantation* 6:83–90, 1968.

192. Blashke J, Severson CD, Goeken NE, et al: Microgranulocytotoxicity. *J Lab Clin Med* 90:249–258, 1977.

193. Lalezari P, Driscoll AM: Ability of thrombocytes to acquire HLA specificity from plasma. *Blood* 59:167–170, 1982.

194. Sharma B, Terasaki PI, Mickey M: Lymphocyte transformation induced by human granulocytes. *Transplantation* 20:499–502, 1975.

195. Thorsby E, Albrechtsen D, Hirschberg H, et al: MLC-activating HLA-D determinants: Identification, tissue distribution and significance. *Transplant Proc* 9:393–400, 1977.

196. Dunstan RA, Simpson MB, Sanfilippo FP: Absence of specific HLA-DR antigens on human platelets and neutrophils, abstracted. *Blood* 64:85a, 1984.

197. Pruzanski W, Farid N, Keystone E, et al: The influence of homogeneous cold agglutinins on polymorphonuclear and mononuclear phagocytes. *Clin Immunol Immunopathol* 4:277–285, 1975.

198. Biberfeld B, Biberfeld D, Wigzell H: Antibodies to surface antigens of lymphocytes and lymphoblastoid cells in cold agglutinin positive sera from patients with *Mycoplasma pneumoniae* infection. *Scand J Immunol* 5:87–95, 1976.

199. Archer GT, Kooptzoff O: Blood group antigens in white cells. *Aust J Exp Biol Med Sci* 36:373–382, 1958.

200. Marsh WL, Oyen R, Nichols ME: Studies of MNSsU antigen of leukocytes and platelets. *Transfusion* 14:462–466, 1974.

201. Marsh WL, Nichols ME, Oyen R, et al: Red-cell blood-group antigens on leukocytes. *Transfusion* 13:343, 1973.

202. Anderson RE, Walford RL: Direct demonstration of A, B and Rho (D) antigens on human leukocytes. *Am J Clin Pathol* 40:239–245, 1963.

203. Marsh WL, Oyen R, Nichols ME: Chronic granulomatous disease and the Kell blood groups. *Br J Haematol* 29:247–262, 1975.

204. Marsh WL: The Kell blood groups and their relationship to chronic granulomatous disease, in Steane EA (ed): *Cellular Antigens and Disease*. Washington, DC: American Association of Blood Banks, 1977, pp 52–66.

205. Marsh WL, Uretsky SC, Douglas SD: Antigens of the Kell blood group system on neutrophils and monocytes: Their relationship to chronic granulomatous disease. *J Pediatr* 87:1117–1122, 1975.

206. Marsh WL: Studies on the Kell blood group system. *Med Lab Tech* 32:1–18, 1975.

207. Marsh WL, Oyen R, Nichols ME: Kidd blood group antigens of leukocytes and platelets. *Transfusion* 14:378–381, 1974.

208. Pierce SR: A review of erythrocyte antigens shared with leukocytes, in Bell CA, (ed): *A Seminar on Antigens on Blood Cells and Body Fluids*. Washington, DC: American Association of Blood Banks, 1981, pp 50–96.

209. Marsh WL, Oyen R: Demonstration of the Gerbich determinants on neutrophil leukocytes. *Vox Sang* 29:69–72, 1975.

210. Kline WE, Press C, Clay ME, et al: Three sera defining a new granulocyte-monocyte-T-lymphocyte antigen. *Vox Sang* 50:181–186, 1986.

211. Van Leeuwen A, Eernise JG, van Rood JJ: A new leukocyte group with two alleles: Leukocyte group five. *Vox Sang* 9:431–446, 1964.

212. Lawler SC, Shatwell HS: A study of anti-5b leuco-agglutinins. *Vox Sang* 13:187–193, 1967.

213. Warren RP, Storb R, Thomas ED: Detection of the leukocyte group-5 on normal and leukemic lymphocytes with the antibody-dependent cell mediated cytotoxicity assay. *Tissue Antigens* 17:174–178, 1981.

214. Van Kessel AHMG, Stoker K, Claas FHJ, et al: Assignment of the leucocyte group five surface antigens to human chromosome 4. *Tissue Antigens* 21:213–218, 1983.

215. Madyastha PR, Glassman AB, Levine DH: Incidence of neutrophil antigens on human cord neutrophils. *Am J Reprod Immunol* 6:124–127, 1984.

216. Warkentin PI, Clay ME, Kersey JH, et al: Successful engraftment of NA1 positive bone marrow in a patient with a neutrophil antibody, anti-NA1. *Hum Immunol* 2:173–184, 1981.

217. Richards KL, McCullough J: Chemotactic and chemokinetic responsiveness of fresh and stored human granulocytes, abstracted. *J Cell Biol* 95:324a, 1982.

218. Gallin JI, Seligmann BE, Fletcher MP: Dynamics of human neutrophil receptors for the chemoattractant fMet-Leu-Phe. *Agents Actions* 12:290–308, 1983.

219. Zola H, McNamara P, Thomas M, et al: The preparation and properties of monoclonal antibodies against human granulocyte membrane antigens. *Br J Haematol* 48:481–490, 1981.

220. Mulder A, Alexander S, Engelfriet CP, et al: Characterization, by immunoprecipitation, of myeloid- and monocyte-specific antigens present on the human promyelocytic cell line (HL-60) in three stages of differentiation. *Proc Natl Acad Sci* 78:5091–5095, 1981.

221. Civin CI, Mirro J, Banquerigo ML: My-1, a new myeloid-specific antigen identified by a mouse monoclonal antibody. *Blood* 57:842–845, 1981.

222. Knapp W: Monoclonal antibodies against differentiation antigens of myelopoiesis. *Blut* 45:301–308, 1982.

223. Perussia BB, Trinchieri G, Lebmand D, et al: Monoclonal antibodies that detect differentiation surface antigens on human myelomonocytic cells. *Blood* 59:382–392, 1982.

224. Skubitz KM, Zhen Y, August JT: A human granulocyte-specific antigen characterized by use of monoclonal antibodies. *Blood* 61:19–26, 1983.

225. Strauss LC, Stuart RK, Civin CI: Antigenic analysis of hematopoiesis. I. Expression of the My-1 granulocyte surface antigens on human marrow cells and leukemic cell lines. *Blood* 61:1222–1231, 1983.

226. Strauss LC, Skubitz KM, August JT, et al: Antigenic analysis of hematopoiesis: II. Expression of human neutrophil antigens on normal and leukemic marrow cells. *Blood* 63:574–578, 1984.

227. Graziano RF, Voll ED, Fanger MW: The expression and modulation of human myeloid-specific antigens during differentiation of the HL-60 cell line. *Blood* 61:1215–1221, 1983.

228. Van Kessel AG, Tetteroo P, van Agthoven T, et al. Localization of human myeloid-associated surface antigen detected by a panel of 20 monoclonal antibodies to the Q12-qter region of chromosome 11. *J Immunol* 133:1265–1269, 1984.

229. Melnick DA, Nauseef WM, Root RK, et al: Monoclonal antibodies (MAB) which inhibit opsonized zymozan (Z) triggered respiratory burst of human polymorphonuclear leukocytes (PMN), abstracted. *Clin Res* 31:370a, 1983.

230. Fleit HB, Wright SD, Unkeless JC: Human neutrophil Fc receptor distribution and structure. *Proc Natl Acad Sci* 79:3275–3279, 1982.

231. Von dem Borne AEGKr, Tetteroo PAT, Bos MJE, et al: Recognition of granulocyte antigens by monoclonal antibodies. *18th Cong Int Bl Transf* 22–27th July, Munich, abstracted. S31-05, 1984.

232. Mulder A: *Myeloid- and Thromobocyte-specific antigens: Studies With Immunofluorescence and Immunoprecipitation*, thesis. Amsterdam, 1982.

233. Thompson BS, Darlow B, Stableforth P, et al: Auto-immune neutropenia in an infant. *Postgrad Med J* 54:278–280, 1978.

234. Reijden HJ, von dem Borne AEGKr, Verheught FW, et al: Granulocyte-specific alloantigen loss in chronic granulocytic leukaemia. *Br J Haematol* 43:589–594, 1979.

235. Lalezari P: Alloimmune neonatal neutropenia, in Engelfriet CP, van Logham JJ, von dem Borne AEGKr: *Immunohaematology*. Amsterdam: Elsevier Science Publishers, 1984, pp 179–186.

236. Levine DH, Madyastha P, Wade TR, et al: Neonatal isoimmune neutropenia, abstracted. *Pediatr Res* 16:296A, 1982.

237. Perkins HA, Payne R, Ferguson J, et al: Nonhemolytic febrile transfusion reactions—Quantitative effects of blood components with emphasis on isoantigenic incompatibility of leukocytes. *Vox Sang* 11:478–600, 1966.

238. Brittingham TE, Chaplin H: Febrile transfusion reactions caused by sensitivity to donor leukocytes and platelets. *JAMA* 165:819–825, 1957.

239. Popovsky MA, Abel MD, Moore SB: Transfusion-related acute lung injury associated with passive transfer of antileukocyte antibodies. *Am Rev Respir Dis* 128:185–189, 1983.

240. Dubois M, Lotze MT, Diamond WJ, et al: Pulmonary shunting during leukoagglutinin-induced noncardiac pulmonary edema. *JAMA* 244:2186–2189, 1980.

241. Andrews AT, Zmijewski CM, Bowman HS, et al: Transfusion reaction with pulmonary infiltration associated with HL-A-specific leukocyte antibodies. *Am J Clin Pathol* 66:483–487, 1976.

242. Ward HN: Pulmonary infiltrates associated with leukoagglutinin transfusion reactions. *Ann Intern Med* 73:689–694, 1970.

243. Butler JJ: Chronic idiopathic immunoneutropenia. *Am J Med* 24:145–152, 1958.

244. Logue GL: Felty's syndrome: Granulocyte-bound immunoglobulin G and splenectomy. *Ann Intern Med* 85:437–442, 1976.

245. Moeschlin S, Siegenthaler W, Gasser C, et al: Immunopancyto-penia associated with incomplete cold hemagglutinins in a case of primary atypical pneumonia. *Blood* 9:214–225, 1954.

246. Craddock PR, Hammerschmidt DE, Moldow CF, et al: Granulo-cyte aggregation as a manifestation of membrane interactions with complement: Possible role in leukocyte margination, micro-vascular occlusion, and endothelial damage. *Semin Hematol* 16:140–147, 1979.

247. Jacob HS, Craddock PR, Hammerschmidt DE, et al: Complement-induced granulocyte aggregation. *N Engl J Med* 302:789–794, 1980.

248. Hammerschmidt DE, Harris PD, Wayland JH, et al: Complement-induced granulocyte aggregation in vivo. *Am J Pathol* 102:146–150, 1981.

249. Goldblum SE, Reed WP: Distribution of *Pneumococcus*-induced augmentation of tissue leukostasis in rabbits: Specificity for the pulmonary vascular bed. *J Lab Clin Med* 105:374–379, 1985.

250. Tvedten HW, Till GO, Ward PA: Mediators of lung injury in mice following systemic activation of complement. *Am J Pathol* 119:92–100, 1985.

251. Hammerschmidt DE, Craddock PR, McCullough J, et al: Comple-ment activation and pulmonary leukostasis during nylon fiber fil-tration leukapheresis. *Blood* 51:721–730, 1978.

252. Graw RG, Herzig G, Perry S, et al: Normal granulocyte transfu-sion therapy: Treatment of septicemia due to gram-negative bacte-ria. *N Engl J Med* 287:367–371, 1972.

253. Goldstein JM, Eyre HJ, Terasaki PI, et al: Leukocyte transfusions: Role of leukocyte alloantibodies in determining transfusion re-sponse. *Transfusion* 11:19–24, 1971.

254. Graw RJ Jr, Stout FG, Herzig RH, et al: Granulocyte transfusion trials at the National Cancer Institute in the granulocyte: Function and clinical utilization, in Greenwalt TJ, Jamieson GA (eds): *The Granulocyte: Function and Clinical Utilization.* Progress in Clinical and Biological Research. New York, Alan R. Liss, 1977, pp 267–281.

255. Clay ME, Kline WE: Detection of granulocyte antigens and anti-bodies: Current perspectives and approaches, in Garratty G (ed.):*Current Concepts in Transfusion Therapy.* Arlington, VA: American Association of Blood Banks, 1985, pp 183–266.

256. Veto RM, Burger DR: The identification and comparison of trans-plantation antigens on canine vascular endothelial cells and lymph-ocytes. *Transplantation* 11:374–377, 1971.

257. Claas FHJ, van Rood JJ, Warren RP, et al: The detection of non-HLA antibodies and their possible role in bone marrow graft re-jection. *Transpl Proc* 11:423–426, 1979.

258. Paul LC, van Es LA, van Rood JJ, et al: Antibodies directed against antigens on endothelium of peritubular capillaries in pa-tients with rejecting renal allografts. *Transplant* 27:175–179, 1979.

259. Logue GL, Shimm DS: Autoimmune granulocytopenia. *Ann Rev Med* 31:191–200, 1980.

260. Weetman RM, Boxer LA: Childhood neutropenia. *Pediatr Clin North Am* 27:361–375, 1980.

261. De Alarcon PA, Goldberg J, Nelson DA, et al: Chronic neutropenia: Diagnostic approach and prognosis. *Am J Pediatr Hematol Oncol* 5:3–9, 1983.

262. Harmon DC, Weitzman SA, Stossel TP: The severity of immune neutropenia correlates with the maturational specificity of antineutrophil antibodies. *Br J Haematol* 58:209–215, 1984.

263. Bussel JB, Hilgartner MW: Annotation—The use and mechanism of action of intravenous immunoglobulin in the treatment of immune haematologic disease. *Br J Haematol* 56:1–7, 1984.

264. Bussel J, Lalezari P, Hilgartner M, et al: Reversal of neutropenia with intravenous gammaglobulin in autoimmune neutropenia of infancy. *Blood* 62:398–400, 1983.

265. Pollack S, Cunningham-Rundles C, Smithwick EM, et al: High-dose intravenous gamma globulin for autoimmune neutropenia. *N Engl J Med* 307:253, 1982.

266. Fagiolo E: Platelet and leukocyte antibodies in autoimmune hemolytic anemia. *Acta Haematol* 56:97–106, 1976.

267. Pui C, Wilimas J, Wang W: Evans syndrome in childhood. *J Pediatr* 97:754–758, 1980.

268. Pegels JG, Helmerhorst FM, van Leeuwen EF, et al: The Evans syndrome: Characterization of the responsible autoantibodies. *Br J Haematol* 51:445–450, 1982.

269. Miller BA, Schultz-Beardsley D: Autoimmune pancytopenia of childhood associated with multisystem disease manifestations. *J Pediatr* 103:877–881, 1983.

270. Linker CA, Newcom SR, Nilsson CM, et al: Combined idiopathic neutropenia and thrombocytopenia. *Ann Intern Med* 93:704–707, 1980.

271. Schreiber AD: Systemic lupus erythematosus—Hematological aspects. *J Rheumatol* 7:395–397, 1980.

272. Svec KH: Immunologic and clinical observations of granulocyte-specific antinuclear antibodies. *Arthritis Rheum* 12:165–172, 1969.

273. Abramson SB, Given WP, Edelson HS, et al: Neutrophil aggregation induced by sera from patients with active systemic lupus erythematosus. *Arthritis Rheum* 26:630–636, 1983.

274. Starkebaum G, Price TH, Lee MY, et al: Autoimmune neutropenia in systemic lupus erythematosus. *Arthritis Rheum* 21:504–512, 1978.

275. Logue GL, Silberman H: Felty's syndrome without splenomegaly. *Am J Med* 66:703–706, 1979.

276. Blumfelder TM, Logue GL, Shimm DS: Felty's syndrome: Effects of splenectomy upon granulocyte count and granulocyte-associated IgG. *Ann Intern Med* 94:623–628, 1981.

277. Petersen J, Wiik A: Lack of evidence for granulocyte specific membrane-directed autoantibodies in neutropenic cases of rheumatoid arthritis and in autoimmune neutropenia. *Acta Pathol Microbiol Immunol Scand* 91:15–22, 1983.

278. Vincent PD, Levi JA, MacQueen A: The mechanism of neutropenia in Felty's syndrome. *Br J Haematol* 27:463–475, 1974.

279. Joyce RA, Boggs DR, Chervenick PA, et al: Neutrophil kinetics in Felty's syndrome. *Am J Med* 69:695–702, 1980.

280. Joyce RA, Chervenick PA, Lalezari P: Immune suppression of neutrophil production in Felty's syndrome: Effects of treatment, abstracted. *Blood* 52:150, 1978.

281. Bucknall RC, Davis P, Bacon PA, et al: Neutropenia in rheumatoid arthritis: Studies on possible contributing factors. *Ann Rheum Dis* 41:242–247, 1982.

282. Dancey JT, Brubaker LH: Neutrophil marrow profiles in patients with rheumatoid arthritis and neutropenia. *Br J Haematol* 43:607–617, 1979.

283. Starkebaum G, Dancey JT, Arend WP: Chronic neutropenia: Possible association with Sjogren's syndrome. *J Rheumatol* 8:679–684, 1981.

284. Stevens DL, Everett ED, Boxer LA, et al: Infectious mononucleosis with severe neutropenia and opsonic antineutrophil activity. *South Med J* 72:519–521, 1979.

285. Schooley RT, Densen P, Harmon D, et al: Antineutrophil antibodies in infectious mononucleosis. *Am J Med* 76:85–90, 1984.

286. Kruskall MS, Weitzman SA, Stossel TP, et al: Lymphoma with autoimmune neutropenia and hepatic sinusoidal infiltration: A syndrome. *Ann Intern Med* 97:202–205, 1982.

287. Hunter JD, Logue GL, Joyner JT: Autoimmune neutropenia in Hodgkin's disease. *Arch Intern Med* 142:386–388, 1982.

288. Weitberg AB, Harmon DC: Autoimmune neutropenia, hemolytic anemia, and reticulocytopenia in Hodgkin's disease. *Ann Intern Med* 100:702–703, 1984.

289. Webster ADB, Platts-Mills TAE, Jannossy G, et al: Autoimmune blood dyscrasias in five patients with hypogammaglobulinemia: Response of neutropenia to vincristine. *J Clin Immunol* 1:113–118, 1981.

290. Cooper DS, Goldminz D, Levin AA, et al: Agranulocytosis associated with antithyroid drugs. *Ann Intern Med* 98:26–29, 1983.

291. Press OW, Fingert H, Lott IT, et al: Pancytopenia in mannosidosis. *Arch Intern Med* 143:1266–1268, 1983.

292. Waugh D, Ibels L: Malignant scleroderma associated with autoimmune neutropenia. *Br Med J* 280:1577–1578, 1980.

293. Danielson DA, Douglas SW, Herzog P, et al: Drug-induced blood disorder. *JAMA* 252:3257–3260, 1984.

294. Price TH, Dale DC: The selective neutropenias. *Clin Haematol* 7:501–521, 1978.

295. Murphy MF, Riordan T, Minchinton RM, et al: Demonstration of an immune-mediated mechanism of penicillin-induced neutropenia and thrombocytopenia. *Br J Haematol* 55:155–160, 1983.

296. Snavely SR, Helzberg JH, Bodensteiner DC, et al: Profound neutropenia associated with benzylpenicillin. *South Med J* 76:1299–1302, 1983.

297. Menitove JE, Rassiga AL, McLaren GD, et al: Antigranulocyte antibodies and deranged immune function associated with phenytoin-induced serum sickness. *Am J Hematol* 10:277–284, 1981.

298. Ream RS, Kerr RO: Neutropenia associated with maprotiline. *JAMA* 248:871, 1982.

299. Albertini RS, Penders TM: Agranulocytosis associated with tricyclics. *J Clin Psychiatry* 39:483–485, 1978.

300. Wall JR, Fang SL, Kuroki T, et al: In vitro immunoreactivity to propylthiouracil, methimazole, and carbimazole in patients with Graves' disease: A possible cause of antithyroid drug-induced agranulocytosis. *J Clin Endocrinol Metab* 58:868–872, 1984.

301. Aisenberg AC, Wilkes BM, Harris NL, et al: Chronic T-cell lymphocytosis with neutropenia: Report of a case studied with monoclonal antibody. *Blood* 58:818–822, 1981.

302. Rumke HS, Miedema F, ten Berge IJM, et al: Functional properties of T cells in patients with chronic Tγ lymphocytosis and chronic T cell neoplasia. *J Immunol* 129:419–426, 1982.

303. Linch DC, Cawley JC, Worman CP, et al: Abnormalities of T-cell subsets in patients with neutropenia and an excess of lymphocytes in the bone marrow. *Br J Haematol* 48:137–145, 1981.

304. Callard RE, Smith CM, Worman C, et al: Unusual phenotype and function of an expanded subpopulation of T cells in patients with haemopoietic disorders. *Clin Exp Immunol* 43:497–505, 1981.

305. Starkebaum G, Martin PJ, Singer JW, et al: Chronic lymphocytosis with neutropenia: Evidence with a novel, abnormal T-cell population associated with antibody-mediated neutrophil destruction. *Clin Immunol Immunopathol* 27:110–123, 1983.

306. Melief CJM: The lymphatic leukemias, in Engelfriet CP, van Loghem JJ, von dem Borne AEGKr (eds): *Immunohaematology*. Amsterdam: Elsevier Science Publishers, 1984, pp 301–321.

307. Chan WC, Winton EF, Check IJ: T-cell imbalance in neutropenia of uncertain etiology. *Am J Clin Pathol* 81:54–61, 1984.

308. Zacharsk LKR, Elveback LR, Linman JW: Leukocyte counts in healthy adults. *Am J Clin Pathol* 56:148–150, 1971.

309. Lichtman MA: Classification of neutrophil disorders, in Williams WJ (ed): *Hematology*, 3rd ed. New York: McGraw-Hill, 1983, pp 770–772.

310. Cutting HO, Lang JE: Familial benign chronic neutropenia. *Ann Intern Med* 61:876–887, 1964.

311. Morley AA, Carew JP, Baikie AG: Familial cyclical neutropenia. *Br J Haematol* 13:719–738, 1967.

312. Lonsdale D, Deodhar SD, Mercer RD: Familial granulocytopenia and associated immunoglobulin abnormality. *J Pediatr* 71:790–801, 1967.

313. Shwachman H, Diamond LK, Oski FA, et al: The syndrome of pancreatic insufficiency and bone marrow dysfunction. *J Pediatr* 65:645–663, 1964.

314. Murdoch JMcC, Smith CC: Infection. *Clin Haematol* 1:619–644, 1972.

315. Arneborn P, Palmblad J: Drug-induced neutropenias in the Stockholm region 1976–1977. *Acta Med Scand* 206:241–243, 1979.

316. Pisciotta V: Drug-induced agranulocytosis. *Drugs* 15:132–143, 1978.

317. Wright DG, Dale DC, Fauchi AS, et al: Human cyclic neutropenia: Clinical review and long-term follow-up of patients. *Medicine* 60:1–13, 1981.

318. Wiseman BK, Doan CA: Primary splenic neutropenia: A newly recognized granulopenic syndrome, closely related to congenital hemolytic icterus and essential thrombocytopenia purpura. *Ann Intern Med* 16:1097–1117, 1942.

319. Amorosi EL: Hypersplenism: *Semin Hematol* 2:249–285, 1965.

320. Ackerman BD: Dysgammaglobulinemia: Report of a case with a family history of a congenital gamma globulin disorder. *Pediatr* 34:211–219, 1964.

321. Blume RS, Bennett JM, Yankee RA, et al: Defective granulocyte regulation in the Chediak-Higashi syndrome. *N Engl J Med* 279:1009–1015, 1968.

322. Miller ME, Oski FA, Harris MB: Lazy leucocyte syndrome: A new disorder of neutrophil function. *Lancet* 1:665–669, 1971.

323. Cordano A, Placko RP, Graham GG: Hypocupremia and neutropenia in copper deficiency. *Blood* 28:280–283, 1966.

324. Al-Rashid RA, Spangler J: Neonatal copper deficiency. *N Engl J Med* 285:841–843, 1971.

325. Mant MJ, Faragher BS: The hematology of anorexia nervosa. *Br J Hematol* 23:737–749, 1972.

326. Warren MP, Vande Wiele RL: Clinical and metabolic features of anorexia nervosa. *Am J Obstet Gynecol* 117:435–449, 1973.

327. Glaser K, Limarzi LR, Poncher HG: Cellular composition of the bone marrow in normal infants and children. *Pediatrics* 6:789–824, 1950.

328. Zuelzer WW, Bajoghli M: Chronic granulocytopenia in childhood. *Blood* 23:359–374, 1964.

329. Bradley PP, Warden GD, Maxell JG, et al: Neutropenia and thrombocytopenia in renal allograft recipients treated with trimethoprim-sulfamethoxazole. *Ann Intern Med* 93:560–562, 1980.

330. Fitchen JH, Koeffler HP: Cimetidine and granulopoiesis: Bone marrow culture studies in normal men and patients with cimetidine-associated neutropenia. *Br J Haematol* 46:361–366, 1980.

331. Muller M, Neftel K, Walti M, et al: Semisynthetische Penicilline und Cephalosporine hemmen die in vitro Myelopoiese dosisabhangig. *Schweiz Med Wochenschr* 113:1471–1473, 1983.

332. Irvine AE, Morris TCM, Kelly GJ, et al: Ticarcillin-induced neutropenia corroborated by in vitro CFU-C toxicity. *Acta Haematol* 70:364–368, 1983.

333. Ascensao JL, Flynn PJ, Slungaard A, et al: Quinidine-induced neutropenia: Report of a case with drug-dependent inhibition of granulocyte colony generation. *Acta Haematol* 72:349–354, 1984.

334. Ellrodt AG, Murata GH, Riedinger MS, et al: Severe neutropenia associated with sustained-release procainamide. *Ann Intern Med* 100:197–201, 1984.

335. Mamus SW, Burton JD, Groat JD, et al: Ibuprofen-associated pure white-cell aplasia. *N Engl J Med* 314:624–625, 1986.

336. Freed N: Idiopathic autoimmune neutropenia: Report of a case. *J Am Osteopath Assoc* 82:419–425, 1983.

337. Hurd, ER, Cheatum DE: Decreased spleen size and increased neutrophils in patients with Felty syndrome: Effects of gold sodium thiomalate therapy. *JAMA* 235:2215–2217, 1976.

338. Hurd ER, Andreis M, Ziff M: Phagotosis of immune complexes by polymorphonuclear leucocytes in patients with Felty's syndrome. *Clin Exp Immunol* 28:413–425, 1977.

339. Wimer BM, Sloan MM: Remission of Felty's syndrome with long-term testosterone therapy. *JAMA* 223:671–673, 1973.

340. Gupta RC, Robinson WA, Kurnick JE: Felty's syndrome: Effect of lithium on granulopoiesis. *Am J Med* 61:29–32, 1976.

341. Messner HA, Fauser AA, Curtis JE, et al: Control of antibody-mediated pure red-cell aplasia by plasmapheresis. *N Engl J Med* 304:1334–1338, 1981.

342. Abdou NI, Verdirame JD, Amare M, et al: Heterogeneity of pathologic mechanisms in aplastic anemia: Efficiency of therapy based on in-vitro results. *Ann Intern Med* 95:43–50, 1981.

343. Novak R, Wilimas J: Plasmapheresis in catastrophic complications of idiopathic thrombocytopenic purpura. *J Pediatr* 92:434–436, 1978.

344. Branda RF, Tate DY, McCullough JJ, et al: Plasma exchange in the treatment of fulminant idiopathic (autoimmune) thrombocytopenic purpura. *Lancet* 1:688–690, 1978.

345. McCullough J, Quie PG: Granulocyte, in Greenwalt TJ, Steane EA (eds): *Clinical Laboratory Science*. Boca Raton, FL: CRC Press, 1981, 1–20.

346. Ambrus CM, Ambrus JL: Regulation of the leukocyte level. *Ann NY Acad Sci* 77:455–486, 1959.

347. Cline MJ: *The White Cell*. Cambridge, MA, Harvard University Press, 1975.

348. McAfee JG, Thakur ML: Survey of radioactivity agents for in vitro labeling of phagocytic leukocytes. I. Soluble agents. *J Nucl Med* 17:480–487, 1976.

349. Weiblen BJ, Forstrom L, McCullough J: Studies of the kinetics of indium–111-labeled granulocytes. *J Lab Clin Med* 94:246–255, 1979.

350. Thakur ML, Segal AW, Louis L, et al: Indium-111-labeled cellular blood components: Mechanism of labeling and intracellular location in human neutrophils. *J Nucl Med* 18:1022–1026, 1977.

351. Thakur ML, Lavender JP, Arnot RN, et al: Indium-111-labeled autologous leukocytes in man. *J Nucl Med* 18:1014–1021, 1977.

352. Weiblen BJ, McCullough J, Forstrom LA, et al: Kinetics of indium-111-labeled granulocytes, in Thakur ML, Gottschalk A (eds): *Indium-111 Labeled Neutrophils, Platelets, and Lymphocytes*. New York: Trivirum Publishing Company, 1980, pp 23–32.

353. Hellum KB, Solberg CO: Human leucocyte migration: Studies with an improved skin chamber technique. *Acta Pathol Microbiol Scand* 85:413–423, 1977.

354. Zakhireh B, Thakur ML, Malech HL, et al: Indium-111 labeled human polymorphonuclear leukocytes: Viability, random migration, chemotaxis, bactericidal capacity, and ultrastructure. *J Nucl Med* 20:741–747, 1979.

355. Alexanian R, Donahue DM: Neutrophilic granulocyte kinetics in normal man. *J Appl Physiol* 20:803–807, 1964.

356. Segal AW, Arnot RN, Thakur ML, et al: Indium-111-labelled leucocytes for localization of abscesses. *Lancet* 2:1056–1058, 1976.

357. Dutcher JP, Schiffer CA, Johnston GS: Rapid migration of
     [111]Indium-labeled granulocytes to sites of infection. *N Engl J Med*
     304:586–589, 1981.

358. Frick MP, Henke CE, Forstrom LA, et al: Use of ^{111}In-labeled leu-
     kocytes in evaluation of renal transplant rejection: A preliminary
     report. *Clin Nucl Med* 4:24–25, 1979.

359. Asher NL, Ahrenholz DH, Simmons RL, et al: Indium 111 autolo-
     gous tagged leukocytes in the diagnosis of intraperitoneal sepsis.
     Arch Surg 114:386–392, 1979.

360. McAffee JG, Gagne GM, Subramanian G, et al: Distribution of leu-
     kocytes labeled with In-111 oxine in dogs with acute inflammatory
     lesions. *J Nucl Med* 21:1059–1068, 1980.

361. Haseman MK, Blake K, McDougall IR: Indium 111 WBC scan in
     local and systemic fungal infections. *Arch Intern Med* 144:1462–
     1463, 1984.

362. Loken MK, Forstrom LA, McCullough, J: 111-indium labeled leu-
     kocytes for diagnosing inflammatory disease of the abdomen and
     retroperitoneal space, in *Radiation and Cellular Response*. Report
     of the Second John Lawrence Interdisciplinary Symposium on the
     Physical and Biomedical Sciences, Sioux Falls, South Dakota, June
     3–4, 1984. Ames, IA: Iowa State University Press, 1983.

363. Lightsey AL, Chapman RM, McMillan R, et al: Immune neutrope-
     nia. *Ann Intern Med* 86:60–62, 1977.

364. Van Rood JJ, van Leeuwen A, Schippers AMJ, et al: Immunoge-
     netics of the group four, five and nine systems, in Curton ES,
     Mattiuz Pl, Tosi RM (eds): *Histocompatibility Testing, 1967*. Balti-
     more: Williams and Wilkins Co., 1967, pp 203–219.

365. Valbonesi M, Campelli A, Marazzi MG, et al: Chronic autoimmune
     neutropenia due to anti-NA1 antibody. *Vox Sang* 36:9–12, 1979.

366. Nepo AG, Gunay U, Boxer LA, et al: Autoimmune neutropenia in
     an infant. *J Pediatr* 87:251–254, 1975.

367. Madyastha PR, Kyong CU, Darby CP, et al: Role of neutrophil an-
     tibody NA1 in an infant with autoimmune neutropenia. *Am J Dis
     Child* 136:718–721, 1982.

368. Kay AB, White AG, Barclay GR, et al: Leukocyte function in a
     case of chronic benign neutropenia of infancy associated with cir-
     culating leukoagglutinins. *Br J Haematol* 32:451–457, 1976.

369. Carmel R: An unusual case of autoimmune agranulocytosis with
     total absence of myeloid precursors: Demonstration of diverse
     sources of R binder for Cobalamin in plasma and secretions. *Am J
     Clin Pathol* 79:611–615, 1983.

370. Sabbe LJM, Claas FHJ, Langerak J, et al: Group specific auto-im-
     mune antibodies directed to granulocytes as a cause of chronic be-
     nign neutropenia in infants. *Acta Haematol* 68:20–27, 1982.

Glossary of Abbreviations

ABC = Avidin-biotin complex (immunoassay)

ACD = Acid citrate dextrose

ADCC = Antibody-dependent cell-mediated cytotoxicity

ADLG = Antibody-dependent lymphocyte-mediated granulocyte cytotoxicity

Af = Antigen frequency

AHG = Antihuman globulin

AIHA = Autoimmune hemolytic anemia

AIN = Autoimmune neutropenia

ANC = Absolute neutrophil count

ANN = Alloimmune neonatal neutropenia

ATP = Autoimmune thrombocytopenic purpura

B-cell = B lymphocyte

BRAB = Bridged avidin-biotin complex (assay)

BSA = Bovine serum albumin

CBC = Complete blood count

CFU-C = Colony-forming unit—culture

CFU-GM = Colony-forming unit—granulocyte macrophage

CIC = Circulating immune complexes

CPD-A1 = Citrate phosphate dextrose—Adenine 1

cpm = Counts per minute

CSA = Colony-stimulating activity

Cyto-B = Cytochalasin-B

DF³²**p** = Diisopropyl phosphofluoridate
DMSO = Dimethyl sulfoxide

EBV = Epstein Barr virus
EDTA = Ethylenediaminetetracetic acid
ELISA = Enzyme-linked immunosorbent assay
Eos = Eosinophil

Fab = A fragment of an immunoglobulin molecule that is involved with antigen binding
F(ab')$_2$ = The antigen-binding fragment of an immunoglobulin molecule after digestion of the molecule with pepsin
FACS = Fluorescence-activated cell sorter
Fc = A crystallizable fragment of an immunoglobulin molecule which is produced by enzymatic digestion of the molecule with papain
FcR = Fc receptor
FCS = Fetal calf serum
FDA = Fluorescein diacetate
FITC = Fluorescein isothiocyanate
fMLP = Formyl-methionyl-leucyl-phenylalanine

GA = Granulocyte agglutination (assay)
GC = Granulocyte cytotoxicity (assay)
GIF = Granulocyte immunofluorescence (assay)
GRS = Granulocyte resuspension solution

HBSS = Hank's balanced salt solution
HLA = Human leukocyte antigen

IEP = Immunoelectrophoresis
IV = Intravenous
IVIg = Intravenous immunoglobulin

k = Kappa (immunoglobulin light chain)
K-cell = Killer-cell (lymphocyte)

λ = Lambda (immunoglobulin light chain)
LAB = Labeled avidin-biotin (assay)
LC = Lymphocytotoxicity (assay)
LRP = Leukocyte-rich plasma
Lymph = Lymphocyte

MCA = Microcapillary agglutination assay
M/E = Myeloid-to-erythroid (ratio)

Mono = Monocyte

n = Number studied
NA = Not applicable
ND = No data
NR = Not reported
NT = Not tested

OD = Outer diameter

p = Gene frequency
p value = Measurement of statistical significance
P = Fisher's exact statistic
PBS = Phosphate-buffered saline
PFA = Paraformaldehyde
PHS = Pooled human sera
PLAST = Neutroplast
plt = Platelet
PMN = Polymorphonuclear leukocyte
PRP = Platelet rich plasma

r = Correlation coefficient statistic
R = Recovery
RBC = Red blood cell
RFI = Relative fluorescence intensity

SD = Standard deviation
SDS = Sodium dodecyl sulfate
SLE = Systemic lupus erythematosus
SPA = Staphylococcal protein A

t½ = Half-life
T-cell = T lymphocyte
TRIS = Tris (hydroxymethyl) aminomethane (buffer)
TRITC = Tetramethylrhodamine isothiocyanate

WBC = White blood cell

Index

Numbers in *italics* refer to pages on which plates, tables, or illustrations appear. Numbers in **boldface** refer to pages on which procedures appear (the number of the procedure is shown in parentheses).

A

ABH antigens, 43, 58–59

Absorption methods for antibody monospecificity, 40, 139
  for antigen cell line distribution, 69, 138–39, **201–4(3.2)**
  using granulocytes, 131–33, **201–2(3.2-A)**
  using platelets (*See* Platelets, absorption method)

ADCC tests, 7

ADLG tests, 6, 24–26, 39, 43, 48, 100, 106, 120–123, **190–95(2.5)**

Agglutination. *See also* Granulocyte agglutination assay
  of leukocytes caused by sera, 3
  phase of granulocyte agglutination (GA) assay, *13–14*

Alleles, dominant, recessive, and codominant, 74

Alloantibodies
  autoantibodies versus, 49–50, 133
  clinical problems due to, 83–90
  directed against blood cells other than granulocytes, identification of, 76–77

Alloimmune neonatal neutropenia (ANN), 4, 5, 47, 52, 54, 65, 112, 200

as a clinical problem due to alloantibodies, 83–85
case study of, 130–31
specimen requirements for, *152*

American Red Cross Blood Services, 153

Aminopyrine
  associated with drug-related granulocyte agglutinating antibodies, 38
  as cause of severe neutropenia in normal patient, 102

Anti-A, Anti-B, Anti-A,B as factors in granulocyte antibody assays. *See* Antibodies, interfering factors in assays of granulocyte

Antibodies. *See also* Granulocyte antibodies
  absorption and elution methods for, 199–206
  characterization of granulocyte, 47–50
  characterization of unknown, 75–81, 136–40
  circulating, 12–28
  cold-reacting, 39–40
  detection of, 5–32, 168–95
  determination of monospecificity of unknown, 40, 139
  drug-related, 3, 38–39, 109
  fluorescent labeling patterns associated with different, 18

interfering factors in assays of granulocyte, 25, 43–45, 151
lymphocytotoxic (HLA) (*See* Human leukocyte antigen system, antibodies)
monoclonal, 44, 59, 67
opsonic, 38
platelet-specific, 77
preservation of granulocyte, 40–41
red blood cell, 76
serologic characteristics of, 48–*49*

Antibody-dependent cell-mediated cytotoxicity (ADCC) tests, 7

Antibody-dependent lymphocyte-mediated granulocyte cytotoxicity (ADLG), 6, 24–26, 39, 43, 48, 100, 106, *120–123*, **190–95(2.5)**

Anticoagulant mixture to maintain granulocyte viability, 151

Antigenic modulation, 29

Antigens. *See also* Granulocyte antigens
  ABH, 43, 58–59
  defined by cold-reacting antibodies, 57
  granulocyte. *See* Granulocyte antigens
  granulocyte-erythrocyte, 60–62
  granulocyte-monocyte-lymphocyte, 62–63

Family studies, 73–75, 130–31, 137–38

Fc receptors, 24, 29, 44

Febrile transfusion reactions, 3, 4, 20, 47, 54, 86–87
case study of, 125–27

Felty's syndrome, 23, 25, 99–100, 112

Fibrin clots, 41

Ficoll-Hypaque gradient, 7–12, **157–59(1.1)**

5a, 5b, 63

Flow cytofluorometry
to analyze fluorescence-labeled cells, 26–27, *66*
for detection of granulocyte-associated immunoglobulin, 30
preparation of granulocytes for, 185

Fluorescein isothiocyanate (FITC), 17, 19, 30, 180–190

Fluorescence-activated cell sorters (FACS), 26

Formyl-methionyl-leucyl-phenylalamine (fMLP) receptors, 66

Functional assays, 6, 20, 28

G

Genetics of granulocyte antigens, 71–81
characterization of new specificities in the, 75–81
exclusion of antigens defined by rare antisera in the, 81
family studies, 73–75, 130–31, 137–38
population studies, 71–73, 136

Granulocyte immunofluorescence (GIF) assay, *17–18, 38–39, 43, 44, 48, 120–123, 149, 150,* **180–90(2.4)**

Gold salts, response of neutropenia with Felty's syndrome to, 112

Gold thiomalate
involved in drug-related immune granulocytopenia, 102
involved in suspected instances of drug-induced neutropenia, 38

Gradients, 7, 9–12

Granulocyte
absorption method for, **201–2(3.2-A)**
cellular destruction of, 105–6
properties of, 5

cytoplasts (neutroplasts), 34–37
for flow cytofluorometry and electron microscopy, 185
indium 111-labeled, 114
in vivo study using a skin window with, 114–15, **222–30(6.2)**
isolation of, 7–12, 28–29, **157–62(1.1, 1.2)**, 164, 169, 174, 178, 181–82, 187, 191–93
kinetics and localization using indium 111, *115–18,* **214–22(6.1)**
preservation, 33–37
production and life span, 113
survival and localization in vivo, 113–24
transfusions, role of antibodies in, 20, 47, 88–89
typing, 135, 151

Granulocyte agglutination (GA), 6, 12–14, *149,* **168–71(2.1)**
antibody class, *48–49*
antibody detection using the, 12–14, *149–150*
applications of the, 4
detection of cold-reacting antibodies with, 39
detection of HLA antibodies with, 43
granulocyte kinetics and the, *120–123*
schematic representation of the, *13*

Granulocyte antibodies, 71
case study of multiparous woman with unidentified, 136–41
characterization of, 47–50
clinical significance of, 83–112
detection methods for, 5–31, 110–11, *150,* 168–98
direct testing for, 28–30
elution of, 37, **204–6(3.3)**
immunochemical characteristics, 47–48
interfering factors in detection of, 43–45
in vitro effects on granulocytes, 5
preservation of, 40–41
specimen requirements for direct testing of, 29
resources required for testing of, 145–147
specimen requirements for detection of, *152*
testing protocol for, *110,* 148–53

Granulocyte antigens, 51–63, 71. *See* Granulocyte-specific antigens
cell line distribution of, 69, 80–81
characterization of, 65–69
clinical significance of, 83–112
disease association, 68–69
expression of, 65–66
frequency in a population, 71–73
frequency of occurrence of, 78–80
gene frequency of, 72
genetics of, 71–81
immunochemistry of, 67
inheritance of, 74, 78–80
nomenclature for N series, 52
phenotypic association with, 77–78
relationship of zygosity and strength of expression of, 67-68
relationships with known antigens, 72–73
"serologically defined" systems of, 6
testing for soluble, 40

Granulocyte-associated immunoglobulin, detection of, 28–31, 44

Granulocyte-erythrocyte antigen(s)
Duffy, 62
Gerbich, 62
HTLA, 62
I/i, 61
Kell, 61–62
Kidd, 62
Lewis, 61
MN, 61
P, 61
Rh, 61

Granulocyte kinetics. *See* Indium 111

Granulocyte-monocyte antigen(s)
AYD, 58
HGA-1, 57–58

Granulocyte-monocyte-lymphocyte antigens, 62–63

Granulocyte-platelet-lymphocyte antigens, 63

Granulocyte serology
evolution of, xv
historical perspectives on, 3–4

Granulocyte-specific antigen(s), *53. See* N series antigens
defined by cold-reacting antibodies, 57

GA, GB, and GC as, 56
Gr, 56
groups 1, 2, and 3, 57
groups 1, 2, 3, 4, and 5, 57
HGA-3, 56
maturation and differentiation, 56
NA, 52–53
NB, 54
NC, 54–55
ND, 55
NE, 55
9a, 54, 55–56
Granulocytotoxicity assay. *See* Complement dependent granulocyte cytotoxicity

H

Haptens, drugs as, 38, 102
Hardy-Weinberg law, 72
Heat inactivation of serum, effect on granulocyte antibodies, 41
Historical perspectives on granulocyte serology, 3–4
Hodgkin's disease, *91*, 96, 100
Human leukocyte antigen (HLA) system, 3, 12
  antibodies, 25, 43–44, 54, 77, 93, *122*, 129, 148–*151*
  antigens, 38
  matching for granulocyte transfusions, 88–89
  matching for kinetics and localization studies, *120–23*
  microlymphocytotoxicity assay for detection of, **195–98(2.6)**
  reactivity, methods for eliminating, 37–38, 148–49, **199–201(3.1)**, **202(3.2-C)**
  stripping, 37–38, 44, **212(5.1)**
  as systemic antigen, 60
  tests for the, in family genetic studies, 77

I

Ibuprofen associated with inhibition of marrow growth, 111
Idiopathic granulocytopenia, immune complexes in patients with chronic, 44
IgG fraction, isolation of, **207–8(4.1)**
IgM fraction, isolation of, **208(4.2)**
Imipramine and granulocytopenia due to bone marrow toxicity, 103

Immune complexes
  in ADLG, 25
  interference in granulocyte antibody assays, 25, 44–45
  role of, in autoimmune neutropenia, 104–5
Immune deficiency diseases associated with granulocytopenia, 101
Immunochemical characteristics of granulocyte antigens and antibodies, 47–48, 67
Immunoelectrophoresis (IEP) to determine immunoglobulin class of column fractions, **210–11(4.3-B)**
Immunoenzymatic assay. *See* Enzyme-linked immunosorbent assay (ELISA)
Immunofluorescence technique. *See also* Granulocyte immunofluorescence (GIF) assay
  for granulocyte antibody detection, 6, 29
Immunoglobulin
  binding methods for granulocyte antibody detection, 6, 16–24, 29–30
  class of column chromatography fractions, determination of, **209–11(4.3)**
  isolation of serum IgG fraction, **207–8(4.1)**
  isolation of serum IgM fraction, **208(4.2)**
Immunoproteins bound in vivo, identification of, 30–31
Indirect granulocyte immunofluorescence, 182–83, 187–88
Indium 111
  body scans in patients with granulocyte antibodies, *122–24*
  decay factor chart, *230*
  granulocyte kinetic studies, **214–22(6.1)**
  granulocyte kinetics in normal subjects using, *115–16*
  granulocyte kinetics in patients with leukocyte antibodies using, 119–122
  granulocyte localization in normal subjects and patients with inflammation, 116, *117–19*, *123*
  granulocytes labeled with, 59, 114–24

  in vivo half-life of granulocytes labeled with, *115*–16, 119–22, *221*
  in vivo localization of granulocytes labeled with, 116–19, *122–23*
  in vivo recovery of granulocytes labeled with, *115*, 116, 119, *120–22*, 218–21
  in vivo studies, 214–30
  leukocyte antibodies studied with, *119–24*
  skin window studies of granulocytes labeled with, **222–30(6.2)**
Infection
  granulocytes localized at sites of, 5
  types of, in patients with primary AIN, 91, 97
Infectious mononucleosis, 39, 100
Inheritance of granulocyte antigens, 74, 140
Inhibition of granulocyte phagocytosis, 6, 28
Inhibition of myeloid maturation, 6, 28

J

Juvenile autoimmune neutropenia, 45, 68–69. *See also* Autoimmune neutropenia (AIN)

K

Killer (K) cells, 24, 25
Kinetic studies. *See* Indium 111

L

Laboratory aspects of primary autoimmune neutropenia, *94–95*
Laboratory space required for granulocyte serology testing, 145
"Leukoagglutination" technique, 3, 12, 86
Leukoagglutinins in sera of polytransfused persons, 3
Leukocyte antibodies
  drug-related, 3
  effect on the fate of granulocytes in vivo of, *119–24*
  role of, in febrile transfusion reactions, 3
Levaminsol
  autoantibodies associated with

granulocytopenia demonstrated in patients receiving, 38
granulocytotoxic autoantibodies occurring in patients receiving, 103

Linkage, determining the probability of, 75

Lithium, response of neutropenia with Felty's syndrome to, 112

"Lod" (log of odds), 75

Lymphatic malignancies associated with autoimmune granulocytopenia, 100–101

Lymphocyte(s)
absorption method using, **204(3.2-E)**
isolation in ADLG, 191–93

Lymphocytotoxicity. *See* Microlymphocytotoxicity test

M

Mannosidosis and autoantibody formation, 101

Maprotiline associated with granulocytopenia, 103

Mart antigen, 62–63, 140

"Maturation arrest" of bone marrow, *94–95*, 111

Methimazole
involved in drug-related immune granulocytopenia, 102
involved in suspected instances of drug-induced neutropenia, 38, 103

Micro method of granulocyte immunofluorescence assay, **180–85(2.4-A)**

Microagglutination tests, 6, 12, **168–71(2.1)** *See also* Granulocyte agglutination assay

Microcapillary agglutination assay, 6, 14

Microgranulocyte cytotoxicity assay, **171–75(2.2)**. *See also* Complement dependent granulocyte cytotoxicity method

Microlymphocytotoxicity (LC) test
for human leukocyte antigen (HLA) antibody detection, 148–*151*, **195–98(2.6)**
to overcome difficulties of standardizing assays and variability of results, 3, 12

Mimicking autoantibodies, 50

Monoclonal antibodies, 44, 51, 67

Monocytes, absorption method for, **202–4(3.2-D)**

Mononuclear leukocytes, isolation of, 7–9

Monospecific conjugates, 132–33, **134–35(2.4)**

Mycoplasma pneumonia, 39, 98

N

NA1. 52–*53. See also* N series (neutrophil-specific) antigens
AIN, 93, 104–12
ANN, 85
autoantibody, 50
juvenile AIN, 44, 52–53, 68–69

NA2, 37, 52–*53*, 54–55, 68. *See also* N series (neutrophil-specific) antigens
AIN, 104–5
autoantibody, 50
juvenile AIN, 52–53, 68–69

National Headquarters Reagent Production Laboratories, 154

NB1, *53*, 54. *See also* N series (neutrophil-specific) antigens
ANN, 85
heterogeneous expression, 66
immunochemical properties, 67
labeling pattern in GIF, 18

NB2, *53* –54. *See also* N series (neutrophil-specific) antigens

NC1, *53* –56, 68. *See also* N series (neutrophil-specific) antigens

ND1, *53*, 55. *See also* N series (neutrophil-specific) antigens
autoantibody, 47
immunochemical properties, 67

NE1, *53*, 55. *See also* N series (neutrophil-specific) antigens

Neutropenia
alloimmune, 19–20, 83–90
alloimmune neonatal. *See* Alloimmune neonatal neutropenia (ANN)
autoimmune. *See* Autoimmune neutropenia (AIN)
causes of, 83, *84,* 107
cellular functions involved in, 106–7
clinical significance of, 107
cyclic, 108–9
definition of, 107
diagnosis of, 107–9, *110*
drug-induced, 38, 102–4, 109, *152*

drugs associated with, *108*
history taken of patients with, 108
immune complexes in, role of, 104–5
infectious diseases possibly associated with, *108*
juvenile autoimmune. *See* Autoimmune neutropenia (AIN)
laboratory studies on, 109–11
neonatal. *See* Alloimmune neonatal neutropenia (ANN)
systematic approach to the evaluation of, 107–12
T-cell involvement with, 106–7
therapy of, 112

Neutrophil Serology Reference Laboratory, 153

Neutrophils
levels of, in patients with primary AIN, *96*
neutropenia caused by decreased production of or increased destruction of, *84*
neutropenia caused by maldistribution of, *84*

Neutroplasts, 34–37
cryopreservation of, **166–67(1.4)**
preparation of, **162–65(1.3)**

9a, 53–56

Nomenclature for neutrophil antigens, development of the, 52

N series (neutrophil-specific) antigens, *53*
antigen expression and zygosity of the, 67–68
chronic granulocytic leukemia, expression in, 69
GA, 14
GIF, 18
SPA, 20
elution of, 37
expression on cord cells, 65
expression on immature cells, 65–66
immunochemical properties of, 47

O

Opsonic assay, *6*

Organ transplantation and production of granulocyte-monocyte cytotoxins, 89

Ouchterlony double agar diffusion, **209–10(4.3-A)**

pulmonary. *See* Pulmonary transfusion reaction
specimen requirements for, *152*
Transplantation
antibodies in bone marrow, 89
antibodies in organ, 89–90
Tricyclic antidepressant drugs,

granulocytopenia as a complication of, 103
Trimethoprim-sulfamethoxazole present during inhibition of marrow growth, 111
Tube method of granulocyte immunofluorescence assay, **185–90(2.4-B)**

Typing reagents for granulocyte antibody testing, 153–54

V

Vancomycin, involved in suspected instances of drug-induced neutropenia, 38

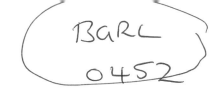

Granulocyte Serology
A Clinical and Laboratory Guide